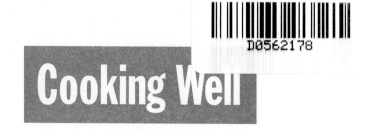

Cooking Well

IBS

Over 100 Easy Recipes for
Irritable Bowel Syndrome
Plus Other Digestive Diseases
Including Crohn's, Celiac, and Colitis

DEDE CUMMINGS
Foreword by Jessica Black, N.D.

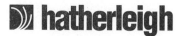

Hatherleigh Press is committed to preserving and protecting the natural resources of the Earth. Environmentally responsible and sustainable practices are embraced within the company's mission statement.

Hatherleigh Press is a member of the Publishers Earth Alliance, committed to preserving and protecting the natural resources of the planet while developing a sustainable business model for the book publishing industry.

This book was edited and designed in the village of Hobart, New York. Hobart is a community that has embraced books and publishing as a component of its livelihood. There are several unique bookstores in the village. For more information, please visit www.hobartbookvillage.com.

DISCLAIMER
This book offers general cooking and eating suggestions for educational purposes only. In no case should it be a substitute nor replace a healthcare professional. Consult your healthcare professional to determine which foods are safe for you and to establish the right diet for your personal nutritional needs.

Library of Congress Cataloging-in-Publication Data is available upon request.
ISBN: 978-1-57826-388-2

All Hatherleigh Press titles are available for bulk purchase, special promotions, and premiums. For information about reselling and special purchase opportunities, please call 1-800-528-2550 and ask for the Special Sales Manager.

Cover and Interior Design by Nick Macagnone
Cover and Interior Composition by DCDesign
Cover Photography by Catarina Astrom (www.catastrom.com)
Photographs on pages 26 and 162 by Samuel C. Carmichael
Photograph on pages 163 and 169 by Lynne Jaeger Weinstein
(www.lynneweinsteinphoto.com)

10 9 8 7 6 5 4 3 2 1
Printed in the United States

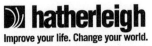

Improve your life. Change your world.
WWW.HATHERLEIGHPRESS.COM

ACKNOWLEDGMENTS

Hatherleigh Press, and the author, would like to extend a special thank you to Jessica Black, N.D.—without your hard work and dedication this book would not have been possible.

The author also wishes to thank the following people for helping this book come to life by sharing recipes, cooking together, and delivering meals when I wasn't feeling well enough to cook. These are friends who really make a difference, especially when one is dealing with a diagnosis like IBS that can be a bit alienating and, at times, debilitating.

Neighbors, and friends, along with some local chefs, and even a writing teacher, all contributed a few recipes to augment my trusty, tried-and-true, hand-written cookbook: Joan Carey, Julie Potter, Suzanne Kingsbury, Teta Hilsdon, Anne Latchis, Johanna Gardner, Orly Munzing (director of the now-legendary Strolling of the Heifers in Southern Vermont), Steve Carmichael, my husband, and my children, Sam, Emma, and Joey. Also, Trina Kassler, Annie Phillbrick, Margy Klaw and her mother, the late Bobbie Klaw, Julie Ewing, Sharon Snider, Carolyn Kasper, John Tobin, Molly Raymond, Lynne Weinstein, Emily Westcott, Laurie Merrigan, Diane Lamb, Connie Cummings, Alex Cummings (and recipe testers, Marcie and Ann Cummings), Steve Rawsome, Christie Herbert, and Renee Lang, N.D., with a special thanks to the long and lasting friendship of Martha Straus, Ph.D.

It is with great pleasure that I also thank my medical and holistic healthcare team: Dr. Steven Bensen, Dr. Horace Henriques, Dr. Jeffrey Potash, Dr. Remeline Damasco, Dr. Laura Metsch, Dr. Wayne Scott Andersen, Dr. Emeran A. Mayer, Samantha Eagle, N.D., Kimberly Timlege, Janet Sinclair, Deborah Feiner-Homer, Heidi Barnes; and I want to thank my CSA (community supported agriculture) farmshare founder of Circle Mountain Farm, Amy Frost. Another big thank you goes to my intern, Taylor Hutcheson, who was a great research assistant and helped by writing a number of drafts throughout this book; the Brattleboro Food Co-op (the caring staff, and especially Julie, Carol, Linda, Charlie, and Susan, in the wellness section),

Dr. Rebecca Jones, Dr. Jennifer Pennoyer, and the local farmers in Southern Vermont. It is a true community that keeps us all healthy!

I want to thank my friend and another Hatherleigh Press author, Kimberly Allison, M.D., author of the forthcoming book, *Red Sunshine*, and director of Breast Pathology at the University of Washington in Seattle. Dr. Allison has been a real inspiration for me and we also share many double tall lattes now on our respective coasts!

In addition, I want to thank a few other friends and authors—Julie Silver, M.D., and Pamela Post-Ferrante. I also want to especially acknowledge the Crohn's & Colitis Foundation of America and my publisher, Andrew Flach, for his unflagging support and for believing in me and my second book. My editorial team was superb: editor Anna Krusinski—along with support from Christine Schultz and Ryan Tumambing—and Carolyn Kasper helped make this book a reality.

—Dede Cummings, author and Crohn's disease patient
who remains in remission for the past 5 years
August, 2011

CONTENTS

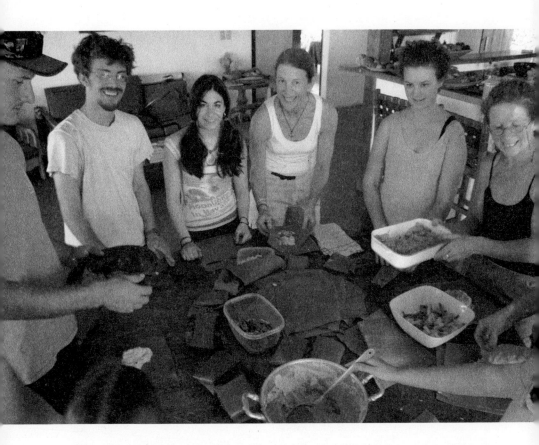

The author (third from right) leads a cooking class in Costa Rica, where the groups she co-leads can travel and spend time learning about the life, food, and culture of Costa Rica (www.cirenas.org).

FOREWORD

"To keep the body in good health is a duty . . .
otherwise we shall not be able to keep our mind strong and clear."

—BUDDHA

To lead a healthy lifestyle, we must consider our relationship with food to be a vital part of survival. If we exist because of the nutrients we consume, our health is reflected by what we eat on a daily basis. There are many important aspects to consider when fueling the body. In current society, our understanding of food for survival and health has declined over generations. Processing and handling has changed our relationship with food and has even altered our taste for food. We have become accustomed to the buttery, rich, sweet flavors of processed foods and the more we eat these types of foods, the more we crave them. Our hunger becomes insatiable when we eat processed, unnatural foods. Obesity and weight gain plague our population, thus contributing to many chronic illnesses. If only the way we ate gave our bodies a better sense of satiety, we could feed our bodies without overeating.

Many generations prior, individuals had to hunt and gather to obtain food. In addition, the food they ate was of utmost freshness and was extremely nutrient-dense, without the added calories, sugar, and fat contained in the foods we eat today.

Earlier generations also experienced stress very differently from the stress we face today. Years ago, stressors were consistently related to survival and were often met with physical demands. In this sense, stress was important because it provided individuals the chemicals needed to move to a safer location or run after their hunt. Due to our present-day sedentary habits and because stress is consistently related to symptoms and flare-ups of digestive disorders, finding ways to reduce stress is essential to digestion and long-term wellness for *all* sufferers.

Earlier in history, when we had to hunt or grow our own food, we appreciated its worth and its gift to us as life-giving power. We were mindful as we shared this food together with our families. It is my assumption that if we once again had to roam, hunt, and gather to obtain food, our culture would be much more appreciative of the food we consume and we would take the time to appreciate the eating process. We can learn something important from indigenous cultures; to honor and cherish the earth for producing our food and allowing us to be nourished. A simple prayer or reflection before meals can change the intent during a family meal. Concentrate on keeping calm, chew your food slowly, and pay attention to the food you are eating. Taking the time to do this during family meals can change how you digest.

It is presumptuous to assume that we can return to those times of hunting and gathering. However, as a society, we can make large efforts to pay more attention to our eating and lifestyle habits. Lifestyle habits can make the difference between disease and wellness. From food choices, exercise, and meal-time habits to meditation and giving thanks, we can make differences in our health, no matter what plagues us.

Serendipity—when two people meet on the street and know they were meant to be there at that precise time in order to meet each other. To know that coming together for them meant something so much more than the sideward glance they shared before enlightenment. In many ways, I feel that my meeting Dede Cummings has been serendipitous.

In working with Dede Cummings, I have learned about the grace and beauty she encompasses in her approach to health and wellness. What Dede suggests in *Cooking Well: IBS* is about simplifying foods and engaging in more meditative habits; practices that our society as a whole has nearly forgotten. My history with Dede suggests a kind of sweet serendipity that catapulted us forward into co-authoring a book together. Our energetic "meeting" really started when Dede's doctor gave her a copy of my book, *The Anti-Inflammatory Diet and Recipe Book*. After using it and enjoying it, Dede contacted me and asked if we could write a book together. We decided to work on it, but with both of our busy schedules, the idea was slowly pushed to the back of my mind as I carried on through my daily life. Then a few years later, Dede announced she had everything ready to go for us to begin writing and we began the incredible journey of working on our first book together, *Living with Crohn's and Colitis* (I say "first book" because I envision us working in tandem for years to come).

Through the process of transferring the manuscript back and forth over thousands of emails, we found that our views on health, meditation, lifestyle, and diet paralleled each others without challenge, even though we had never met. So, actually our serendipitous meeting was at a book signing after we had already finished our manuscript together!

In *Cooking Well: IBS*, Dede does a wonderful job of simply bringing us through IBS and other digestive disorders, and improving our understanding of the medical thought process behind diagnosis. Interestingly, Dede was wrongly diagnosed with IBS, which often happens when someone suffers from gastrointestinal problems without a discoverable cause. Dede has such an accessible and personal writing style that brings you into a more positive state of mind. You may find yourself thinking, "I can do that" or, "I really am going to feel better." This is a powerful part of healing. A person cannot heal if he or she doesn't believe it. Many of my patients with the best attitude, good sense of humor, balanced lifestyle, and affinity for exercising are the patients that get well the quickest.

It is extremely important to consider that our relationship with food will affect how we heal. Food is central to the entire chasm of living beings. Practically, food provides nutrients for our body's fuel. It is central to more than you may be aware of. Food stimulates conversations, initiates friendships and relationships, pleases customers, and praises employees. Food is *everywhere*. Think of how often you may have scheduled a social activity that involved food in one way or another. Dates, having people over, parties, ceremonies, going out after work, going to a friend's house for dinner, lunch meetings, breakfast meetings—these are just a few examples of the many ways that we interact with each other around food.

So why is it that societal food choices are not typically healthy and nourishing? We have veered far from our roots in our food choices and farming practices. Research has shown that poor food choices affect health outcomes for the future. There is a direct correlation between fats, sugars, and processed foods and illness. There is also a direct relationship between healthy foods such as vegetables, fruits, nuts, seeds, and other high-fiber foods and a decrease in negative health outcomes. It is being proven in the research, now we just need to start listening and making changes in our own lives.

As hard as change is, it can be liberating and exhilarating. Increasing healthy foods in your diet is a good start and Dede has done a great job of presenting us with delicious recipes in a way that enables us to still savor food, without having to sacrifice taste.

I am positive that you will be thanking yourself for picking up this book and will enjoy putting into practice some of the suggestions that Dede offers in the following pages.

—Jessica Black, N.D.
Author of *The Anti-Inflammatory Diet and Recipe Book*
and co-author of *Living with Crohn's and Colitis*
www.afamilyhealingcenter.com
www.herb-fusion.com

Chapter 1

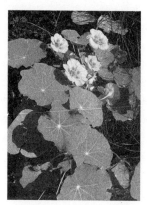

Living with IBS

Irritable bowel syndrome (commonly referred to by lay- and medical personnel alike as IBS) is a condition occurring in the large intestine that causes cramping, bloating, gas, diarrhea, and/or constipation for a short period of time. These symptoms usually clear up on their own without the aid of medication, and adjusting one's diet is an effective way to aid in recovery from a flare-up of IBS, and keep symptoms from recurring.

IBS is known in the medical world as a functional disorder, which means exactly what it sounds like: the organ does not function properly. Sometimes it is even hard to function enough to do simple things like travel, or socialize, due to the discomfort.

As is the case with many digestive diseases, doctors are not sure what causes IBS—some people report feeling cramps or have diarrhea during a meal and have to be excused to go to the bathroom; others report discomfort after the meal, as the food is moving down into the digestive tract.

Regardless of the lack of definitive causes, it is important to note that the word "syndrome" connotes a variety of symptoms and the reason they appear has not been made clear to the physician. The patient usually reports his or her symptoms and it is the doctor who then looks for the cause. An actual set of disease characteristics is often vague in IBS and the disease's pathophysiology (by definition, the functional changes associated with or resulting from disease) cannot be determined.

In medicine, a mechanical-physical, or body-biochemical problem can be analyzed and summed up as a type of disease using pathology; however a disease that presents with a cluster of sometimes-unrelated symptoms, like those of IBS, makes it harder to diagnose. Oftentimes the patient complains of ancillary, or secondary, symptoms like headaches and body aches or pains that may or may not be linked.

Dede's Experience

During my own initial struggles with IBS, my general practitioner had a hard time trying to figure out what was the matter with me. I kept complaining about feeling anxious, having stress in my life, and being worried about the failing health of my father. All of these factors made it hard for my doctor to pinpoint exactly what was going on, especially with the added emotional stress and problems I described, that kept cropping up.

My doctor did, however, diagnose the loosely-named IBS in my case, and sent me home with very little medication to alleviate my group of symptoms: cramping, occasional diarrhea with sudden onset, trouble sleeping, and headaches and irritability.

Symptoms of IBS include:
- Diarrhea
- Cramping
- Gas
- Bloating
- Constipation
- Overall abdominal pain
- A mucus discharge mixed with bowel that is whitish
- A swollen, somewhat distended belly
- For women, sometimes symptoms increase during menses

Causes of IBS

Irritable bowel syndrome is not even characterized as a disease; rather it is within a hard-to-classify group of symptoms that is difficult to pin down. The short answer is that doctors don't really know what causes IBS. Perhaps the muscles of the large colon don't contract or expand properly to aid in the digestion of food; or, rather than a mechanical problem, the patient has trouble breaking down food due to an overly-sensitive gut that is prone to cause gas and bloating.

The causes of inflammation for those with IBS and other forms of more complicated cases of Inflammatory Bowel Disease (IBD) are complex, involving a number of factors. These include one's environment, microbial balance, genetics, stress and emotional health, diet and lifestyle habits, and immunological factors.

IBS and Stress

Current medical research looks at the biological effects of sleep and exercise on mood, affect, and wellbeing in the field of IBS. Stress neurobiology is a specific area being studied at UCLA in the NIH-funded UCLA Center for Neurobiology of Stress, Division of Digestive Diseases. Dr. Emeran Mayer's research focuses on the ancient practices of yoga and meditation as having the potential for healing modalities that reduce stress and encourage overall health and healing.

As many of us are aware, stress has a significant and impressionable influence on all diseases. In fact, stress and the hormones that are secreted in times of excess stress directly affect our aging. In today's world, our lifestyles play a huge role in the prevalence of particular diseases, including all chronic illnesses and cancer.

Stress is a controversial cause of IBS because there are conflicting studies on the relation of stress and IBS. However, when we look at the picture of IBS through pathophysiology and clinical experience, it is clear that stress is absolutely connected to IBS. Stress may not be the *cause* of IBS, but it is certain that many with the syndrome report their symptoms and condition worsen when under stress. If you have IBS and are reading this text, you can most certainly attest to what is being suggested. Haven't you spent more time in the bathroom when you are under extreme stress? Or before you have to give a presentation at work, or a lecture, or some other important event, do you ever feel "butterflies in your stomach," as the old saying goes?

Any chronic illness brings with it the complexities of the mind/body connection. Ways to de-stress in one's life can be easy, but like most things, require patience and practice. The following chapters will include a few tips to guide one who suffers from the myriad of symptoms related to IBS. The recipes have been chosen to offer a range of choices that one can use as a preventative measure to encourage overall health, especially through a low-inflammation diet.

Treatment for IBS

When a doctor suspects IBS, he or she will order a round of basic tests to rule out other diseases, like ulcerative colitis or Crohn's disease (which fall into another digestive disease category called Inflammatory Bowel Disease/ IBD). A test called a colonoscopy is a way for the doctor to look inside the large intestine (and usually most of the small intestine) to examine the delicate lining and make sure there are no polyps or irritations along the lining of the colon.

In addition to blood work and a physical examination, some doctors will order a stool sample, but this is not typically done because the tests take time and are expensive—many naturopathic doctors like to spend as much time as possible determining just what the symptoms arise from. Traditional physicians have a hard time keeping up with their immense patient caseloads and may refer the patient to a naturopath who is trained to take a more holistic approach. Either way, a full medical history is important.

Overall Tips for Better Digestive Health and Wellness

Improve your diet. The very first change that should occur in patients wanting to improve their health is a dietary change. Even minor dietary changes can affect health significantly and usually larger dietary changes can bring even better results. Diet is extremely important to health. Try avoiding processed foods and foods with additives, colors, and preservatives. Avoid sugars, especially items sweetened with refined sugars such as high-fructose corn syrup.

Make lifestyle changes. Changing your lifestyle can be liberating and engaging. It can enable you to become more aware of your body and any changes that are occurring, as opposed to merely taking a drug and waiting for the symptom to disappear. Integrating whole-body treatment and lifestyle changes can help to improve overall health rather than focusing on one issue or one specific problem. One important lifestyle change to make is creating a routine and rhythm for yourself. Go to bed at the same time, get up at the same time, and eat meals at the same time. Routines promote better breathing and consistency in diet, sleep, and exercise, which creates better health and better resistance to illness.

Begin an exercise routine. Exercise is one of the most important lifestyle practices to begin when considering treatment options. No matter what your physical state, there is always something you can do for exercise. Following a daily plan is essential to maintaining good health. If you currently don't have an exercise program, try walking first. Thirty minutes to one hour of walking outside can help improve mood and energy.

Maintain a holistic approach to your health. Taking supplements, getting a stool sample analysis, and going to a psychotherapist, massage therapist, or naturopathic physician are all effective starting points to building an overall holistic treatment plan that achieves results for patients suffering from IBS.

Increase socialization in your life. Laughter is extremely important for emotional and physical health. Laughter, along with socializing with friends and joining a support group through your local hospital or naturopathic health clinic, can really be beneficial in helping relieve stress. Online social media communication is helpful as well, but real-time interactions are always best.

Increase body awareness. For an entire week, try writing in a journal all the symptoms you experience and everything you are doing and eating. Be sure to record all symptoms, from the most minor crick in the neck to low back pain, headaches, or diarrhea. By doing this, you can learn how your body is trying to communicate with you, how you can listen to your body, and what changes you can make, if needed.

Try yoga or meditation. Meditation is an extremely important, yet very simple, relaxation tool. Yoga is a great way to relax and is most effective by adopting a regular routine. Try a DVD at home or you can join a class with a trained yoga teacher.

What About Other Digestive Diseases?

This cookbook will also aid those suffering from other forms of inflammation-related diseases, not just IBS. The recipes are specific to aiding in digestion, especially when the immune system is compromised, with the outcome to lower inflammation and create a balance of sustenance that will help create an overall digestive plan to follow. The use of olive oil, fresh vegetables, wild-caught fish, and organic food overall (made without being processed or fried) is the basic foundation for health. Specific recipes, such as Fish Curry on page 72, are loaded with natural immune boosters in the spices, and protein from the fish, which can be used by those readers who suffer from Crohn's, ulcerative colitis, or celiac disease.

When one is diagnosed with a condition such as rheumatoid arthritis, multiple sclerosis, chronic fatigue syndrome, diverticulitis, or GERD (gastroesophageal reflux disease), it can be a daunting task to navigate daily life. Since inflammation in one's diet can affect joints and one's entire digestive tract, it makes sense to eat the most balanced, and healthiest, diet.

Following the instructions on lifestyle and diet outlined in this book will also empower patients, or caregivers, to take necessary steps to eliminate inflammation in the diet and lower stress to more manageable levels.

Dede's Experience

In my daily life, I try to eat the freshest, least-processed foods available, and the "localvore" movement is a way to participate on a community level. By "localvore" I mean food that is grown and produced within a 50-mile radius of where you live; food that is not shipped from foreign countries whereby losing nutritional value. According to one of my favorite authors, Michael Pollan, "If it came from a plant, eat it; if it was made in a plant, don't" (*Food Rules: An Eater's Manual,* Penguin, December 29, 2009, 27). In Pollan's book, he recommends a plant-based diet, and stresses the importance of avoiding processed and overly-refined foods. These are certainly wise words to live by.

Chapter 2

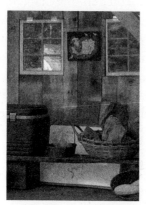

How the Right Diet Can Help

Although there is no dietary "cure" for IBS, eating well can make a major difference for those living with the symptoms. Choosing the right foods and avoiding the wrong ones can help reduce (and possibly eliminate) the occurrence of symptoms and lead to a more normally functioning digestive tract.

By shifting to an IBS-friendly diet, the body will not only be receiving rich nutrients, but will also become more regulated, allowing the digestive tract muscles to relax and easily break down the food.

Increasing the intake of the right fruits, vegetables, grains, and meats while staying away from fatty, sugary, and stomach-straining foods, can lead to better well-being with less symptoms and more time to just be you. This will also hopefully keep your health on track for years to come.

Making the Right Choices

The dietary suggestions outlined in this chapter will help create a meal plan that will steer clear of the IBS "trigger" foods, which can be a setback on the quest for a healthy and symptom-free diet.

Keep in mind that each individual is different and not everyone will have the same reactions to certain foods. However, some people will prefer to eliminate all foods that characteristically worsen symptoms.

Speak to your doctor about the dietary guidelines below and seek his or her guidance based on your own unique symptoms and needs before beginning any dietary regimen.

Basic Nutrition

If you haven't already, omit from your daily diet any foods that irritate or increase your IBS symptoms; this can drastically improve your digestive health and regularity. These dietary changes can be your first step towards better health:

- **AVOID** dairy products like milk, cheese, and yogurt. Even if you're normally tolerant to these foods, the high fat content can lead to diarrhea and increase digestive discomfort.
- **AVOID** certain vegetables like broccoli, Brussels sprouts, cabbage, and cauliflower, which increase gas.

  Note that excessive intake of fiber can also lead to gas and cramping. However, depending on your symptoms, a gradual increase of soluble fibers (such as apples, oats, and citrus fruits) and insoluble fibers (found in whole grains, bran, and most vegetables) can help relieve constipation by moving material through the digestive system.
- **AVOID** artificial sweeteners and foods high in sugar.
- **AVOID** red meat and fried, fatty, and processed foods.
- **ALSO AVOID** caffeine, alcohol and chocolate.

Keep in mind that it will take time to eliminate any food products that you are accustomed to using. By using the trial and error system (and documenting the results in a food journal) you can rule out certain foods that have a negative effect on your specific symptoms.

Dede's Experience

People always ask me why I can't eat wheat, and I don't have a clear answer. I remember my naturopath asking me to give up wheat when I was having digestive issues—mostly constipation and blockages—and I was horrified. "I love pizza and bagels the most," I pleaded with her. She demurred and suggested I give up wheat for three days to see if that helped my frequent bouts of arthritis (a result of long-term Crohn's disease).

After three days, I was ecstatic. I had more energy, and I felt better all over, especially in my elbows and knees which were frequently arthritic. Five years have now passed, and I switched to the ancient wheat grain, Spelt, for my occasional wheat-fixes (though I typically use rice flour for pastas and pizza crusts). Spelt looks very similar to wheat—just ask my seventeen-year-old son who often samples my Spelt concoctions, like pizza dough and scones, and doesn't notice any difference from the same made with wheat! Spelt actually contains more protein than wheat, and since I eat very little red meat, I do like getting extra protein in my diet. In addition, the protein is easier to digest; however, there is actually more gluten in Spelt, which makes it an unsuitable grain for those with celiac disease.

These basic guidelines can also help you when creating a regulated diet schedule:

- **Keep up nutrients:** Eliminating certain food groups like dairy, which provides calcium and potassium, can be replaced by taking adequate supplements so that your body can still receive the benefits of those vital nutrients.
- **Eat often:** Eating small meals throughout the day on a routine schedule will help increase regularity. Large meals can strain the digestive flow, thereby increasing symptoms like constipation and/or diarrhea.
- **Eat slowly:** Eating in a relaxed environment and taking time to savor your meals can help reduce sudden gas, bloating, and diarrhea or constipation.
- **Stay hydrated:** Increase your intake of liquids throughout the day, especially water. This can decrease the amount of bloating and gas.
- **Relax and rest:** Resting after meals will slow the digestive process, which reduces the sudden onset of diarrhea and/or constipation.

Dede's Experience

There is a great deal of discussion on whether drinking, say, eight glasses of water per day, is helpful; again, each person is different, and it is worth noting in your food journal whether drinking water really makes a difference for you. I know when I travel on airplanes, I get very dehydrated due to the stale air and cabin pressure—I sometimes even get mild migraine headaches when I am dehydrated. To help alleviate this, I carry a water bottle with me at all times, and I drink many additional glasses of naturally-sweetened cranberry juice and soda water made using our "at home" carbonated water mixes (see the References Section on page 163 for details on this device and others).

Dietary Suggestions

Specific foods and herbs can especially help IBS patients. In addition to following the basic guidelines listed above, these items can help regulate and decrease symptoms:

Eat foods high in potassium. Especially if you have diarrhea, your body can lose electrolytes. Fish, nectarines, potatoes, nectars, and avocados are high in potassium and will re-boost electrolyte levels.

Drink herbal teas that promote good digestion. Herbal teas like catnip/fennel, peppermint/spearmint, wild yam, chamomile, and thyme help with digestion and rid the colon of fermenting waste, which will relieve pain.

Knowing your body and your individual symptoms will help create a diet that is suited just for you. Since IBS symptoms can vary widely from case to case, there is no universal right and wrong when it comes to dietary choices. There are foods that can increase diarrhea but may soothe constipation and vice versa. Being aware of your personal restrictions will be most beneficial in short-term relief.

Following these guidelines can help reduce the frequency of diarrhea:
- Limit your fat intake; replace fried foods with cooked or baked meals and try low-fat versions.
- Reduce spicy foods, which can cause digestive flare-ups.
- Rest after meals to slow digestion.

- Avoid foods that cause gas (see Basic Nutrition on page 12)
- Limit high-fiber foods like beans and nuts.

Following these guidelines can help reduce the frequency and severity of constipation:
- Increase fiber intake; beans, nuts, whole-grains, and bran.
- Drink plenty of water.
- Loosen stools with the sugar sorbitol, found in prunes and prune juice (take in moderation as to not cause diarrhea).
- Avoid caffeinated drinks, which cause dehydration.

Dede's Experience

When my symptoms are acting up, I resort to what is known as the BRATY diet, until the symptoms start to ease up. BRATY is an acronym for the following foods: bananas, rice, applesauce, toast, and yogurt. This is a tried-and-true method of mine (and many others) that eases the stress on my digestive system and quiets things down. Since everyone is different, there may be substitutions (for instance, I do not eat wheat, so I eat bland rice cakes instead).

Eating Well: Making a Change

Keeping a food journal is really important for sufferers of IBS, both young and old. A food journal is a great way for young IBS patients to feel more stable as it can also include anecdotes of the child's day, complete with pictures.

The journal can be a way to focus on the possibility of stressful situations and how to avoid them in the future, including which foods to avoid. It can also point out positive things such as safe foods or helpful and enjoyable experiences.

For an entire week, try writing in a journal all the symptoms your body has and everything you are doing and eating. By doing this, you can learn how your body is trying to communicate with you, how you can listen to your body, and then change if you need to. The more you do this, the easier it will become to notice these connections.

For example, maybe you have diarrhea intermittently but can never relate it to anything. By doing the journal, you may learn that each time you have a double-tall caramel macchiato, you have diarrhea three hours later. If you notice a connection similar to this, then you know that you should do what is right and healthy for your body and stop consuming any foods or drinks that do not agree with your body. Another example would be if you notice that you are constipated each time your period is about to begin. In this case, you may have some problems with hormone regulation and should be evaluated by a naturopathic physician to make sure your hormones and glandular function is occurring optimally.

Dede's Experience

When I first started keeping a food journal, I discovered very quickly that I would need to avoid MSG after having eaten a take-out dinner from a local Chinese restaurant, which was followed by cramps and a mild flare-up.

Keep the Momentum Going

The information presented in this book is not a definitive guide, nor does it present a cure. However, one major equation in overall success is patient participation, and you hold the key to your own best life. Having a positive attitude is key!

During the path to health, it is imperative to focus on adequate nutrition, rest, exercise, water, sunshine, detoxification, along with a positive attitude and expectation for yourself, forgiveness, and appreciation. Such ongoing activities and attitudes are the foundations of health. Remember, the goal is to achieve a balance of lifestyle and digestive wellness. It is difficult to actually ask for help, as everyone wants to be successful and function independently. One way to ask for help is to practice with your friends and loved ones. If you are having a bad day and feel like you need to stay by the bathroom, call a friend, or your spouse, and ask them to pick up some ginger tea, rice crackers, and a movie to distract you. You will be surprised at the results!

Reaching Out

As mentioned above, you will be pleasantly surprised when you reach out to others and ask for help. Take baby steps. For example, if you feel like you don't feel comfortable asking a friend for help, call a church group or a "meals-on-wheels" non-profit agency, and see if you can get some support. Trade with a friend from your support group, if you find one in your area (check the local hospitals for this as many are beginning to offer IBS/IBD support services), and work out a barter. For example, you can say to someone, "I will help you one day a week, or be on call, if you help me."

Talk to your relatives and friends and try to educate them about IBS. Tell them, honestly and without hiding much, how you feel (I know it is hard to talk about diarrhea, but most people will be sympathetic; if not, maybe they should move off your A-list of friends!). It is important that people accept you for who you are, and that you tell them you may need their support for the long haul, and not just for an isolated moment.

Dede's Experience

My friend, Molly, and I often planned potluck dinners together. Even though she now lives far away, we always recall how much fun we had in the process. Her husband had a very restricted diet due to health problems, and I was struggling with a diagnosis of IBS in the 1990s. Molly and I collaborated to bring our two families together with our children participating, too, as we gathered in one of our kitchens to chop, prepare, roast, peel, and blend various savory, locally-grown vegetables and steamed brown rice. We often used wheat-free tamari to spice up the vegetables and served the whole thing over rice with some sautéed tofu (a soy-based, protein-rich food made by coagulating soy milk with resulting curds pressed into soft white blocks—I personally like the firmer blocks—that can be cut into cubes and fried in olive oil and garlic, or steamed with vegetables in a steamer over boiling water), for a delicious dinner!

Don't Forget to Breathe

Making sure to breathe deeply is important for your health. Deep breathing exercises are extremely effective in handling depression, anxiety, and stress-related disorders.

Begin by inhaling through the nose as much as you can, paying attention to the abdomen and making sure it is freely moving and again, repeat the inhalation, with the next deep breath. Do this for at least five complete breaths. If you have time for more, continue this for another minute or so.

Doing this daily breathing technique and making it a habit is the first step in building an exercise program, if you are not already doing so. You will likely notice a difference fairly quickly after adopting this breathing exercise daily. Rodney Yee's *AM/PM Yoga* video leads you through gentle yoga stretches to guided meditation—yoga/meditation practice has been proven to help relieve stress.

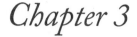

Chapter 3

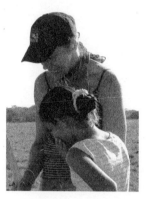

Dietary Suggestions for a Healthy Lifestyle

E ating well should be a top priority, no matter what your fitness level or what your age or health status. You have a responsibility to your body to maintain good health and keep up a stable and beneficial diet. Taking responsibility for this diet is a daily task, and not necessarily an easy one, but staying on track with your eating goals will lead to the overall health you deserve. Always pay attention to your nutrition plan and do everything in your power to stay as close to it as possible.

Keep in mind that there will be days that you veer off course—this is understandable. Changing your eating habits is a big adjustment; breaking these habits may mean straying from many years' worth of cultural and family habits. Be realistic and honest with yourself; accept that this is a process and that change won't happen overnight. A strong will is a must; no change will occur unless you commit yourself to seeing it happen. By staying optimistic and on-track with your dietary needs, this transitional process will be easier.

Maintaining a healthy diet is not about eating everything you like, and it may require sacrificing some of your less-healthy favorites. Healthy eating is about providing your body with the foods it needs. It is about eating the right amount of calories per day considering your daily activities. It is about helping yourself in the long-run by eating the foods and adapting to the habits that will keep you lively and pain-free.

Eating healthy is also about meal rituals. That means having regular meals at the same times every day. Especially for those suffering from IBS symptoms, scheduled eating times can be extremely beneficial. It is recommended that you eat smaller, more frequent meals throughout the day instead of three or four large meals. You can decide what works for you individually—in many cultures it is customary to walk after a meal, which serves as an aid to digestion! Make sure to always listen to your body, acknowledge your symptoms, and create the appropriate change that will allow your digestive system to function more regularly.

Remember that eating should also be a pleasant experience, and eating well doesn't have to be a daunting task. Fresh fruits and vegetables as well as lean, locally-raised, and organic meats (or wild-caught and sustainably-harvested fish), when eaten plain or in a delicious recipe, can brighten your day.

Eating Organic

According The Organic Center (www.organic-center.org) located in Boulder, Colorado, eating organic foods improves the overall health for the earth and its inhabitants. This is a pretty strong statement, and one that we all should fully support. Through research, education, farming, and purchase of organic fruits, vegetables, fish, poultry, and meat, we can all partner together to attain the healthiest goals possible. Results from this wonderful center show that organic foods are able to deliver more nutrition per calorie than their non-organic counterparts.

According to the Center's website, "'Certified Organic' means the item has been grown according to strict uniform standards that are verified by independent state or private organizations. Certification includes inspections of farm fields and processing facilities, detailed record keeping, and periodic testing of soil and water to ensure that growers and handlers are meeting the standards which have been set."

Here are a few tips to consider when purchasing organic food:

- Organic frozen food is a great way to purchase healthy foods during the winter when they are not in season.
- You can also buy larger quantities when they are on sale and store in your freezer for a few months without worrying about spoilage (for example, I like to freeze organic blueberries, without even washing them. They freeze really well in zip-lock bag portions, and can be added to pancakes made with gluten-free flour to enhance the flavor and create a healthier breakfast).
- Read food labels carefully—make sure there is no added sugar and that the label shows USDA standards.
- To wash off any bacteria from fruits and vegetables, use a scrub brush to clean and then run under cold water.
- Buy in bulk to save money—you can store root vegetables in a cool place or freeze them (corn, for example, can be shucked and the kernels frozen in zip-lock bags).
- Make sure you buy local and in season as this will ensure the freshest ingredients, and sometimes the cost is lower as there is no middle-broker or mark-up involved.
- In order to buy local as much as possible, ask your local store where the food comes from if it is not noted on the label—more and more shoppers are becoming aware of the "localvore" movement and make it a priority to support local growers.

Support your local farmers and growers. The more distance the food travels from farm to table, the greater the cost. Join a food co-op. Co-ops purchase food in bulk and often carry organic items. If there isn't one in your town, consider starting one with family and friends. Also, look for a local CSA (Community Supported Agriculture) farm stand in your area, where you can shop for local and organic vegetables, free-range chicken eggs, and broiler chickens on a weekly basis. Riding your bike or walking to the farm share is a great way to do the weekly pickups and get some exercise at the same time!

Buy organic meat and chicken from local growers. You can search for local CSA farm shares in your area that raise organic, grass-fed beef or free-running chickens, and you won't need to buy such large portions for each person this way. The nutrients found in fresh, organic meat is far superior than the supermarket shipped-in varieties, so you can justify the extra cost by serving smaller portions.

Another important reason to purchase organic food is to help keep our water supply clean. Agricultural runoff is a major problem in conventional farming methods as herbicides can leak into water supplies and spread contamination. Organic farming methods work to prevent runoff contamination, which is a factor in why it is a forward-looking way of farming as opposed to a fad!

Eating Out

Many restaurants use commercially packaged food and unhealthy fats, which are detrimental to your health. Due to this, you should eat out no more than twice a week. Eating out is a nice treat to look forward to, perhaps on weekends, when you can relax and enjoy being out with family or friends. Although you deserve this carefree time away from the kitchen, make sure not to stray too far from your specific diet. Always make sure that you pay close attention to the type of foods you choose when going out, as to avoid the sudden onset of symptoms.

Many chefs will be willing to prepare your dish how you need it. In order to have a wider variety of suitable and enjoyable choices, choose a restaurant that caters to foods closer to your diet. Don't feel shy about asking your restaurant server about the ingredients in a dish and mention that you are on a specific diet (for example, wheat-free or gluten-free), and ask them for recommendations. Steer clear of staple dishes at characteristically spicy restaurants, as these hot dishes might increase symptoms. Vegetarian, Mediterranean, and seafood restaurants will likely serve a wide variety of safe and delicious options.

> ### Dede's Experience
>
> When I go to a dinner party, I get bombarded with questions about my diet such as, "Why don't you eat wheat?" Or, "Why can't you eat the spicy chicken dish?" People can sometimes be a bit insensitive to those of us with dietary restrictions. If this happens to you, politely tell them that you are undergoing a transformative, life-changing experience that they can participate in if they purchase this book and embark on their own healthy eating plan!

Dede's Tips for Restaurant Ordering

- Drink a tall glass of water before a meal. This will help you feel a bit fuller, and you will be less inclined to snack on chips or anything else that may be on the table and are loaded with salt and possible IBS triggers, like wheat.
- If ordering salad dressing and sauces that might be too spicy for you, ask to have it as a side dish, which will allow you to use sparingly as needed.
- When the server offers the usual "rice, baked potato, or French fries," option, always choose the rice first and the baked potato second.
- Don't eat desserts, unless they offer something like fresh berries. Instead, ask for peppermint tea with honey at the end of a meal.

If you are traveling to a friend's house for a visit, don't be shy about telling them your dietary restrictions—people often shop before visitors arrive, and this way they will feel confident when selecting an alternative for you to eat during your stay. This might also help your host decide on menu items or allow you to prepare an alternative meal for yourself if the food being served will trigger any symptoms. A good rule of thumb is to eat very little, and don't eat anything you have never had before. Social gatherings should not be an excuse to veer off from your daily diet routine. Always make sure you know what is in the food and how it was prepared.

When flying, try the vegetarian or gluten-free alternative meal, ordered in advance, which will probably include less risky ingredients. Even still, ask specifically what foods are included in the meals. Nuts, raisins, carrots, and crackers are easy to carry and you will be able to find bottles of water almost everywhere (I usually try to carry my own water bottle in a stainless steel container which saves unnecessary plastic waste, though this may not always be possible, especially in airports). Make sure to avoid caffeinated drinks, which might seem temporarily helpful when traveling long distances. If you are prone to caffeine-induced symptoms, certain teas like green tea and chamomile will give your body helpful nutrients without upsetting your system.

Basic healthy cooking for IBS, Crohn's disease, and/or ulcerative colitis (not to mention Celiac disease), can be challenging in general, but especially so when on the road. Being able to know your body's tolerance for certain foods is key to planning your diet, and traveling makes it hard to do that. Prior to your trip, and in general, it is a good idea to keep a food journal, as mentioned in Chapter 2.

No one diet is completely right for everyone with IBS or IBD. Keeping a food journal will help you find out which foods cause problems for you. Then you can avoid those foods and choose others that supply the same nutrients, especially while traveling. For example, some people with IBS may have problems digesting legumes, fiber-rich foods, raw salads, spices, additives, preservatives, fried foods, or berries and fruits with seeds.

For those individuals who either are still having significant symptoms or have very sensitive digestion, steaming or cooking most foods (even fruits) can help significantly. By steaming or cooking, it reduces the live enzyme content of the food and makes it significantly easier on your digestion. Make sure to chew foods well and eat slowly. For some, taking two teaspoons of organic apple cider vinegar in a little bit of water before meals can also aid digestion.

Eating healthily and happily involves an investment of time and creativity, but preparation helps make the diet transition go smoothly. There are many techniques to create fast, easy, and healthy meals, even when you travel. For example, you can plan to cook your own dinners a few nights, and include some of your favorite comfort foods like beans and rice, along with local plantains and broccoli.

Dede's Experience: Travel

Most mornings on my recent vacation to the island of Roatán (off the coast of Honduras), I made a green drink to start the day right, with a generous serving of oatmeal and bananas (I have always been able to find oatmeal when I travel, but just in case, I packed a few packets of instant Kashi™ oatmeal as a back-up, though it is normally too sweet for me).

To create healthy meals while on the road, Jessica Black, N.D. and I recommend you use techniques such as steaming, sautéing, puréeing, chopping small, blending, grinding, and many others. If there is a health food store near you or a restaurant that serves healthy meals, go there first, especially as you adjust to a new climate and location.

While on vacation, I ordered fresh fish, rice, and streamed vegetables for practically every meal! In the morning, I had oatmeal with bananas and honey, and would often boil a few eggs to keep in the fridge as a snack. Lunch was mostly corn tortillas with beans and rice: All these foods were "tried and true" in my diet—with a proven track record for wellness in my case (remember how helpful the food journal is!).

In addition, I kept my morning yoga routine and seated meditation—this vacation allowed me to do that on my own private beach, which was a great way to begin the day with sun salutations.

Gone are the days of partying and drinking wild concoctions of Island Rum and piña coladas! However, I did enjoy a light beer made in Honduras, without any problems. I also drank tons of water on the trip, which was especially helpful when flying on airplanes since it tends to dehydrate travelers in general.

Getting lots of restorative sleep was easy—being by the ocean tends to lull one into sleep effortlessly. All-in-all, travel is something us Crohn's and UC patients, as well as those with IBS, can manage with careful planning and knowledge of the food and culture as well.

Some IBS sufferers get constipated while traveling, so it is especially important to take extra fiber (even packets of Metamucil® are helpful, though you should use the sugar-free variety if you can) while you travel.

If you do go to a market, don't forget to wash your vegetables and fruits with a bottle of water mixed with a little vinegar. This will help kill bacteria that may not be visible to the eye. A basic rule of thumb is wash it, peel it, and boil it (or avoid it!). Although much of this may seem daunting, don't forget to enjoy your travels and relax! Having a stress-free trip will greatly benefit your body and naturally improve your mood.

Dede's Experience

I always travel with my little "kit," which is a freezer bag filled with my ground flax seed, probiotic supplement capsules that I get from the naturopath, omega-3 capsules, multi-vitamins, and vitamin C, along with some applesauce and rice cakes (remember the BRATY acronym for bananas, rice, applesauce, toast, and yogurt) to supplement my diet on the road. The wonderful-tasting rice crackers available in stores nowadays are great to snack on and are handy for emergencies when you need some extra nutrition, or something to spread some delicious almond butter on, which is a much healthier alternative to peanut butter.

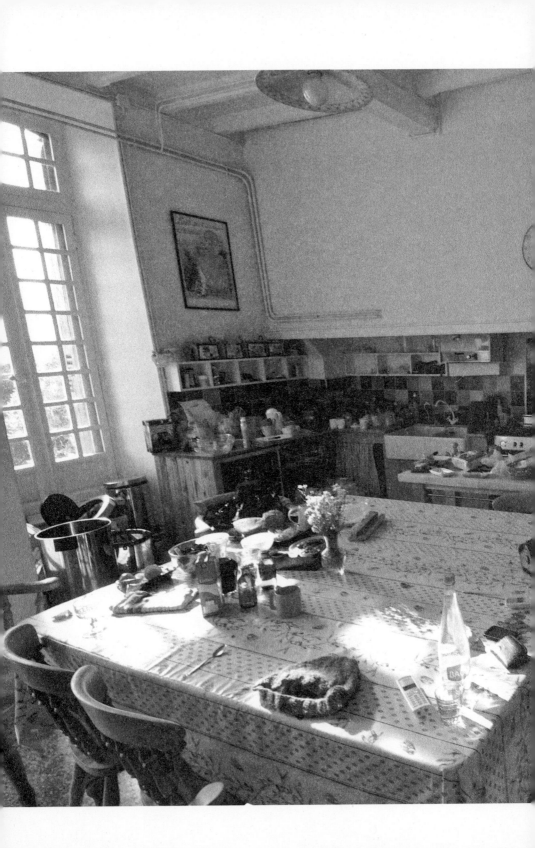

Chapter 4

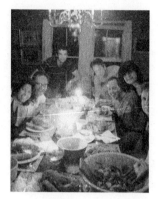

The Recipes

Breakfast

"Instant" Oatmeal Your Way

Serves 1

½ cup water
¼ cup regular oatmeal
1 tablespoon raisins
⅛ teaspoon cinnamon

Place water in bowl. Add oatmeal, raisins, and cinnamon. Stir to combine. Microwave on high for 1½ to 2½ minutes. Cook for the minimum amount of time and check to see if the oatmeal is cooked enough for your taste. If not, continue cooking until desired doneness. Stir after removing from the microwave. Add milk and enjoy!

Other Ideas for Your "Instant" Oatmeal
- Cook with milk instead of water to increase calcium.
- Add fresh, frozen, or canned fruit of your choice. The fruit can be cooked with the oatmeal, but you may prefer to add the fruit to the cereal after it is cooked.
- Use other dried fruits, like cranberries or chopped apricots, in place of the raisins.
- Add 1 tablespoon of peanut butter to oats before or after cooking.
- Add 1 tablespoon of chopped nuts.
- Add 1 teaspoon of honey, maple syrup, brown sugar, etc.—all have approximately 4 grams of carbohydrates per teaspoon.

For more substitution information, please see page 159.

Basic Familia Cereal

Serves 2

1½ cup rolled oats
½ cup rye, wheat or barley flakes
½ cup wheat germ
½ cup raisins
½ cup slivered almonds
½ cup dried, chopped dates, prunes, and/or figs
½ cup sesame seeds
½ cup sunflower seeds
½ cup dried apple slivers
½ cup unsweetened shredded coconut
½ cup non-fat dry milk

Mix all ingredients in a large bowl.

Eat with milk or even add fruit and/or yogurt.

Store, covered tightly, in refrigerator.

Best-Tasting Power Protein Bars

(As seen in *Living with Crohn's and Colitis* by Dede Cummings and Jessica Black, N.D.)

These bars make excellent alternatives for breakfast and snacks on the go. Be careful—these are so good, they're addictive! Also, this recipe tends to vary depending on the liquid content of the almond butter and the quality and texture of the protein powder. You may need to alter the amount of liquid, depending on how the mixture stays together during the hand mixing process.

Makes 1 dozen (Servings dependent on cut size of bars)

1½ cups rice crisp cereal
¼ cup sunflower seeds, half ground
¼ cup pumpkin seeds, half ground
2 tablespoons sesame seeds
2 tablespoons hemp seeds
8 scoops or servings protein powder (whey, soy, rice, or other protein powder alternative)
½ teaspoon sea salt
1½ cups almond butter
1½ cups brown rice syrup

Prepare a greased 9- × 9-inch or 9- × 13-inch baking pan or simply line the pan with two layers of wax paper. In a separate bowl, mix all dry ingredients together. Warm almond butter and brown rice syrup in a saucepan over medium heat until soft and fluid. Pour over dry ingredients and begin working mixture with your hands into a large clump. Thoroughly mix the mixture to evenly coat entire dry mix. Press tightly into greased pan or wax paper lined pan and chill in refrigerator until hard. Once hard, cut into squares and store in airtight container. These can very easily be stored in the freezer and taken out a few hours before enjoying.

Gluten-Free Banana Granola Pancakes

(As seen in *Living with Crohn's and Colitis* by Dede Cummings and Jessica Black, N.D.)

Serves 4

2 bananas, ripe
¾ cup hemp milk
1 teaspoon vanilla extract
½ teaspoon baking soda
½ teaspoon cinnamon
1½ cups gluten-free pancake or baking mix
1 cup granola

Heat lightly oiled skillet to medium heat. Add bananas, milk, and vanilla to blender and blend until smooth. Add baking soda, cinnamon, and half of the baking mix and blend until smooth. Add the second half of the baking mix and blend until smooth. Remove blender, add granola to the mixture and mix in with mixing spoon. Do not blend. Pour batter into 3-inch diameter circles in the pan. When pancakes start to bubble, flip them carefully and cook on the other side until lightly browned on both sides.

Easy Pancakes with Ground Pumpkin and Sunflower Seeds

(As seen in *Living with Crohn's and Colitis* by Dede Cummings and Jessica Black, N.D.)

Serves 4

3 tablespoons ground pumpkin seeds
3 tablespoons ground sunflower seeds
3 organic eggs
¼ cup non-gluten flour
¼ cup hemp milk, or other alternative milk
2 teaspoons baking soda
¼ cup uncooked millet (optional)
¼ cup blueberries (optional)

Heat lightly oiled skillet to medium heat. Combine all ingredients except blueberries and millet into a medium-sized bowl and mix well until clumps have dissolved. Add blueberries and/or millet if you are going to use these ingredients. Pour batter into 3-inch diameter circles in the pan. When pancakes start to bubble, flip them carefully and cook on the other side until lightly browned on both sides.

Blueberry Syrup

(As seen in *Living with Crohn's and Colitis* by Dede Cummings and Jessica Black, N.D.)

This recipe was given to Dr. Black by Cathe Frederick of Grande Rond, Oregon.

Serves 4

2 cups organic blueberries
Stevia, to taste

Take two cups of blended blueberries and strain to remove stems. Cook on low heat and stir frequently to form a light syrup. Cool slightly and sweeten with pure Stevia to taste. Serve over pancakes or light desserts.

Bran Muffins

Makes 1 dozen

¼ cup all-purpose flour
1 tablespoon baking powder
3 tablespoons granular sucralose
½ teaspoon salt
1 cup 100% bran cereal
1 cup skim milk
1 egg
¼ cup vegetable oil
Nonstick spray

Preheat oven to 400°F. Coat a muffin pan with nonstick spray. In a medium bowl, combine flour, baking powder, sucralose, and salt; set aside. In a large mixing bowl, combine cereal and milk; let stand for 2 minutes. Add egg and oil; mix well. Add dry ingredients, stirring just until moistened. Spoon into muffin cups coated with cooking spray. Bake for 18 to 20 minutes or until golden brown. Remove to a wire rack to cool.

Laurie's Fruit Smoothies

Serves 1

1 cup skim milk or non-fat/low-fat plain or flavored yogurt (read nutrition facts label for carbohydrate content)
½ cup fruit, sliced or chopped

Combine ingredients in a blender. Process ingredients until the ingredients are smooth.

If you don't have a blender, use a container with a tight-fitting lid. Mash fruit or chop finely. Put fruit in container. Add milk or yogurt and shake briskly.

Smoothies can also be made using a hand mixer, whisk, or egg beater. Put fruit and milk/yogurt in a bowl and whip until frothy.

Sunny Morning Burrito

Serves 1

¼ cup chopped vegetables (*see note)
1 egg (**see note)
1 (6-inch) tortilla
1 tablespoon salsa (optional)
½ tablespoon light sour cream (optional)

In a small nonstick skillet, lightly sauté the chopped vegetables.
Add the egg, stir to scramble. Cook until dry. Heat tortilla between
wet paper towels for 30 seconds in the microwave. Tortillas can also
be heated in the oven by wrapping in aluminum foil and baking at
350°F for 5 minutes.

Tortillas roll more easily when warm. Fill tortilla with the egg
and vegetable mixture. Serve with salsa or low-fat sour cream, if
desired.

*Leftover vegetables work well in this recipe. Use several kinds of
vegetables (it's okay if you use more than the ¼ cup).

**To reduce cholesterol, replace the egg with an egg substitute or two
egg whites.

Pumpkin-Herb Biscuits

Serves 6

½ cup all-purpose flour
½ cup whole-wheat flour
1½ teaspoons baking powder
2 tablespoons chopped, fresh chives (or 1½ teaspoon dried chives)
¼ teaspoon nutmeg
¼ teaspoon salt
⅛ teaspoon black pepper
2 tablespoons beaten whole egg or egg substitute
¼ cup canned pure pumpkin (not pumpkin pie filling)
¼ cup buttermilk (or skim milk)
1½ tablespoons canola oil
Nonstick spray

Preheat oven to 475°F. Spray a baking sheet with nonstick spray. Combine first 7 ingredients (flour through pepper) in a large bowl. Make a well in center. Beat egg with a fork, in a medium bowl. Add pumpkin, buttermilk, and canola oil. Stir until blended. Add pumpkin mixture to flour mixture. Mix until a dough forms (do not overmix). Turn dough out onto a floured board or work surface. Press into 1-inch thickness. Cut with 2-inch round cutter. Arrange on the prepared baking sheet. Bake for 12 to 15 minutes until golden on top. Serve warm or at room temperature.

Breakfast Apple Pie

Serves 1

1 slice whole-wheat bread
¼ cup applesauce
⅛ teaspoon cinnamon
1 slice low-fat cheese (1 ounce)

Lightly toast the bread. Mix applesauce and cinnamon together.

Spread applesauce on top of toast to the edge of the bread so it won't burn. Top with a slice of cheese. Broil or bake until cheese melts.

Homestyle Cheese Muffins

Makes 1 dozen

2 cups all-purpose flour
3 teaspoons baking powder
½ teaspoon salt
1 egg, slightly beaten
1 cup skim milk
¼ cup margarine, melted
½ cup shredded reduced-fat cheddar cheese
Nonstick spray

In bowl, combine flour, baking powder, and salt. Mix egg, milk and margarine in separate bowl, then mix into dry ingredients, just until moistened. Fold in cheese. Coat muffin cups with cooking spray, then fill two-thirds full.

Bake at 400°F for 20–25 minutes or until golden brown.

Soups & Salads

Winter Squash Soup

Serves 4

2 pounds butternut squash
1 cup water
1 teaspoon salt
1 cup chopped onion
½ clove garlic, minced
2 tablespoons butter
2 cups milk
2 cups light cream (optional)
½ cup cooking sherry
Salt and pepper, to taste
Toasted sliced almonds
Sour cream (optional, to garnish)

Peel, seed, and dice squash. Combine with water and salt in saucepan. Bring to boil and simmer covered until squash is mushy, or at least very tender.

Meanwhile, sauté the onion and garlic in butter until tender. Liquefy squash and onions with milk and cream in blender. Add sherry, salt, and pepper. Heat until hot.

Serve garnished with toasted almonds and/or a generous dollop of sour cream (optional).

Fresh Minestrone

Serves 4

1 onion, chopped
1 garlic clove, crushed
Pinch oregano
1 teaspoon margarine
1 small potato, peeled and diced
1 carrot, diced
¼ pound green beans, diced
1 stalk celery
1 small tomato
Some parsley, chopped
1 small leek (optional)
½ can mushrooms (optional)
½ cup corn (optional)
2 okras, cut (optional)
½ cup zucchini, sliced (optional)
¼ cup cabbage, shredded (optional)

Combine onion, garlic, and oregano with margarine. Cook over low heat until onion is golden. Add 2 cups water and bring to a boil. Add vegetables in order of firmness. Simmer on low heat until vegetables are tender, but still crisp.

Serve in warm soup bowls, thickly garnished with parsley.

This dish is especially good with grated Parmesan cheese and warm garlic bread.

Lentil Apricot Soup

(As seen in *Living with Crohn's and Colitis* by Dede Cummings and Jessica Black, N.D.)

This soup was introduced to Dr. Black by her good friend, Desiree LeFave, a licensed midwife whom she works with often.

Serves 4

3 tablespoons olive oil
1 onion, chopped
2 cloves garlic, minced
⅓ cup dried apricots, minced
1½ cups red lentils
5 cups vegetable broth or chicken broth
½ teaspoon ground cumin
½ teaspoon dried thyme
3 plum tomatoes, peeled, seeded, and chopped
2 tablespoon fresh lemon juice
Salt and ground black pepper, to taste

Sauté onion, garlic, and apricots in olive oil. Add lentils and broth. Bring to a boil, then add spices, reduce heat, and simmer for 30 minutes, covered, and stirring occasionally. Add tomatoes and simmer 10 minutes more. Add lemon juice and puree half of the soup in the blender. Add pureed half back into the soup and serve warm.

Lynne's Curried Lentil Soup

½ cup canola or safflower oil (or butter)
2 yellow onions, diced ¼-inch
4 cloves garlic, chopped
5 carrots, peeled and cut into ½-inch pieces
5 celery stalks, cut into ½-inch pieces
1 teaspoon curry powder, or more to taste
2 cups lentils, rinsed and stones removed
Salt and freshly ground pepper, to taste
Fresh ground ginger, to taste (or 1 can crushed tomatoes), optional

In a heavy stew pot, add oil or butter and sauté onions, add garlic, carrots and celery, and cook until soft. Add curry powder (and either fresh ground ginger or a can of crushed tomatoes, if using), salt, and pepper. Then add lentils and enough water to cover ingredients by an inch. Bring to a boil the turn down heat, let simmer for a hour or more. The longer it cooks, the better it tastes. Add more water if needed. The soup should become thick and mushy—you can puree it in a blender if you choose.

Cold Cucumber Soup

Serves 6–8

3 large cucumbers
½ onion, sliced thin
2 tablespoons butter, unsalted
½ cup bay leaves
1 tablespoon flour
3 cups low-sodium, fat-free chicken broth
1 teaspoon kosher salt
1 cup half-and-half
2 tablespoons lemon juice, fresh or bottled
½ teaspoon dill weed, fresh or dried
1½–2 cups sour cream
Additional dill for garnish

Peel two of the cucumbers. Slice and sauté in butter along with the onions and bay leaves until tender, but not brown. Blend the flour. Add broth stirring until smooth. Add salt and simmer covered, about 25 minutes. Discard bay leaves.

Puree in food processor or blender. Pour through a strainer and discard any solids. Chill well. (The soup can be frozen at this point, or refrigerated for up to 2 days.)

The day of serving; skim off any fat on the surface. Add half-and-half, lemon juice, and dill weed to the chilled mixture.

Peel the remaining cucumber; cut it in half length wise, scoop out the seeds, and coarsely grate. Cover and refrigerate until serving time. This can be done an hour or two ahead.

Place about 1 heaping tablespoon of grated cucumber in the bottom of each bowl. Add soup, a dollop of sour cream.

Chilled Eggplant Soup

Serves 8

¼ cup olive oil
1 large eggplant, peeled and cut into small cubes
1 large green pepper, seeded and chopped
2 garlic cloves, minced
¾ cup water
6 sprigs fresh mint
1 quart plain yogurt
3 tablespoons chives, fresh chopped

Heat the olive oil in a large sauce pot, over medium heat. Add the eggplant, garlic, and pepper and cook for 2 minutes. Add water, reduce heat to medium, and simmer for 15 minutes.

Cool the cooked vegetables until they reach room temperature. Add yogurt and mint to the mixture, and puree in a blender until smooth.

Chill soup for at least 3 hours before serving. Serve cold and garnish with chopped chives and mint sprigs.

Farmers' Market Soup

Serves 6

Stock
1 medium carrot, minced
1 stalk celery, minced
2 medium onions, minced
1 medium shallot, minced
1 medium leek, minced
3 cloves garlic, crushed and unpeeled
7 cups homemade chicken broth (or use low-sodium canned broth)
6 peppercorns
1 sprig fresh thyme
5 parsley stems
Nonstick spray

Soup
2 medium leeks, white and light green parts only, halved lengthwise
    and cut into 1-inch lengths
6 small red potatoes, scrubbed, cut into ¾-inch chunks
1 cup frozen peas, thawed
2 cups packed baby spinach
2 tablespoons chopped fresh parsley leaves
1 tablespoon chopped fresh tarragon leaves
Salt and freshly ground black pepper, to taste

Stock
Completely wash and clean all vegetables used in stock (and
soup). Combine the carrot, celery, onions, shallot, leek, and garlic
in a heavy-bottomed stock pot. Lightly spray the vegetables with
cooking spray, toss, and coat.

Cover and cook the vegetables over medium heat, stirring
until slightly softened and translucent, about 6 minutes. Add the
broth, peppercorns, thyme, and parsley stems. Increase the heat

to medium high and bring to a simmer. Continue until stock is flavorful, about 15 minutes. Strain the stock, discarding solids.

Soup
Bring the stock to a simmer in a large heavy pot over medium heat. Add the prepared leeks and potatoes and simmer until potatoes are tender, about 9 minutes. Stir in pears, spinach, parsley, and tarragon. Season to taste with salt and pepper.

Butternut Parsnip Soup

Serves 4

1 medium-large butternut squash
3–4 parsnips
3 tablespoons olive oil, divided
1 teaspoon salt
1 cup chopped onion
5 cups chicken broth
1 cup apple cider

Preheat oven to 375°F.

Peel squash and parsnips and cut into 1-inch cubes. Toss in 2 tablespoons olive oil and spread on baking sheet. Salt lightly and bake for approximately 30 minutes or until slightly caramelized and soft.

Sauté chopped onion in soup pot with remaining tablespoon olive oil over medium heat for 5 minutes. Add squash, parsnips, chicken broth, and apple cider. Bring to a simmer and cook for about 20 minutes.

Process in a blender, food processor or with a hand-held immersion blender, until smooth.

Robust Chicken Noodle Soup

Serves 2

1 can chicken noodle soup (low-salt variety)
½ to 1 cup leftover vegetables or canned, organic (no-salt-added
   varieties) or frozen vegetables
½–1 cup leftover cooked chicken

Put chicken noodle soup in saucepan. If using a variety that calls
for adding water, do so. Add vegetables and chicken. Heat until
hot. Serve.

Dr. Lang's Healing Soup

Contributed by Renee Lang, N.D.

Serves 4

2 tablespoons miso paste *(enzymes and nutrients)*
1 quart water, filtered *(cleaner and fewer toxins)*
2 cups organic broccoli, chopped *(nutrient content, fiber, and liver support)*
2 cups organic carrots, chopped *(nutrient content, fiber, and liver support)*
1 tablespoon organic ginger, minced *(anti-inflammatory, digestive aid, and liver support)*
4–6 cloves organic garlic, minced *(anti-oxidant, anti-microbial, and liver support)*
⅛–¼ cup tamari, to taste *(enzymes)*
1–2 tablespoons sesame oil *(taste and a little fat to balance the meal)*
1 cup quinoa *(excellent source of protein)*
Onions minced (optional) *(anti-oxidant, vitamin C)*
Turmeric, minced (optional) *(anti-inflammatory, anti oxidant)*
Cilantro, minced (optional) *(excellent detoxifier, chelator of metals)*

Heat water and add miso paste. Do not allow water to boil, but simmer. Allow paste to dissolve.

When dissolved, add broccoli, carrots, ginger, garlic, tamari, sesame oil, and quinoa. Cook until vegetables are tender, about 30–60 minutes.

For easy digestion and optimal absorption, blend the soup. This will break down the broccoli and carrots even further for ease of digestion.

Taste and add tamari or sesame oil as desired for flavor.

For each ingredient, the benefits to a balanced gut have been marked in italics.

Curry Turmeric Leek Soup

Serves 4

3 tablespoons olive oil
2 leeks, sliced
5 cloves elephant garlic, sliced into large slices
½ head Napa cabbage
1 bok choy, chopped
1 quart chicken broth
1 can diced tomatoes
3 teaspoons curry powder or more to taste
1 teaspoon turmeric powder
1 teaspoon fish sauce
½ teaspoon organic lemon juice
Sea salt, to taste

Add olive oil to large saucepan or soup pot on medium low
heat. Add leeks and elephant garlic and sauté until medium soft.
Increase heat to medium and add cabbage and bok choy and sauté
for 3–5 minutes. Then add all other ingredients, cover, and simmer
on medium to low heat until flavors mingle and vegetables are
cooked but still maintain their crunch.

Creamy Avocado and Pea Soup

Serves 6

2½ cups almond milk (see note)
2 cups fresh peas
2 avocados
Sea salt, to taste

Place all ingredients in blender and blend until smooth, adding
more almond milk if desired to adjust thickness.

> If you have a good blender, such as a Vitamix® (see page 165 in the
> References section), you can choose to make your own almond milk
> using raw organic almonds.

Gazpacho

Serves 4

5–6 tomatoes
½ red pepper
½ green pepper
2 garlic cloves
½ onion
¾ cucumber, seeded (about 5–6 inches)
2 tablespoons white vinegar (I use champagne vinegar)
3 tablespoons olive oil

Purée all ingredients.

This can also be heated, but it is best served chilled.

To serve, garnish with chopped onions, cucumbers, and tomatoes.

> This recipe was prepared at my friend, Julie's, home in Washington, DC. She attended the Farmers' Market the morning my flight landed and made the two dishes, which we ate later for lunch—delicious and so easy!

Corn Salad

Serves 4

3–4 ears fresh, local corn
4 tomatoes
1 small bunch fresh basil
12 ounces feta cheese

Steam corn cut off cobs and mix together in a salad bowl with freshly-harvested corn; toss with tomatoes, fresh basil, and feta cheese, then serve.

My friend, Julie, also made this delicious and easy corn salad for our "Girls' Weekend" lunch.

Tabouli

(As seen in *Living with Crohn's and Colitis* by Dede Cummings and Jessica Black, N.D.)

This makes a very pretty dish and is always great to bring to a potluck or celebration meal. If you cannot tolerate tomatoes, try replacing them with chopped cucumbers and Kalamata olives.

Serves 4

1 cup quinoa, cooked and cooled
2 cups filtered water
2 bunches parsley, regular or flat-leaf, minced
1 pint cherry tomatoes, cut in quarters
2–3 cloves garlic, chopped fine
½ cup organic lemon juice
⅓ cup organic cold pressed olive oil
Sea salt, to taste

Start by cooking the quinoa. Add 1 cup of quinoa and 2 cups filtered water to a pan and cover. Bring to boil, reduce heat to medium low, and allow to boil/simmer until all the water has been absorbed. Stir occasionally to keep the quinoa from burning on the bottom of the pan. When all the water has been absorbed, remove from heat and allow to cool.

   Add cooked quinoa, parsley, garlic, and tomatoes into a large bowl. Pour lemon juice, olive oil, and salt over the mixture. Mix well and chill in refrigerator for at least 30 minutes prior to serving.

Chilling for at least 24 hours helps the flavors mingle even better.

Spinach Salad

Serves 4

Dressing
2 tablespoons olive oil
1 tablespoon cider vinegar
1 tablespoon chopped fresh parsley
1 teaspoon lemon juice
1–2 packets sucralose

Salad
1 cup cooked whole-grain bowtie or rotini noodles
2 cups torn raw spinach or salad mix
¾ cup sliced celery
¼ cup sliced green onions
1 medium tomato or 1 cup cherry tomatoes
½ cup raw snow peas
1 cup seedless grapes (optional)
½ pound cooked shrimp or 8-ounce chicken breast (optional)

Dressing
Place all dressing ingredients in pint jar, close with lid, and shake
well.

Salad
Cook noodles according to package directions, but do not add salt
to water. Drain, rinse, and cool. Place torn fresh spinach in large
salad bowl. Chop celery and green onions. Slice fresh tomato into
small wedges or cut cherry tomatoes into halves. Wash grapes and
snow peas and add all to salad bowl.

If using cooked fresh or frozen shrimp, remove peels and veins.
If using cooked chicken, cut into bite-size pieces using separate
cutting board. Add to salad bowl. Place drained and cooled pasta
in salad bowl. Shake dressing and pour over salad. Toss with salad
tongs or 2 large spoons.

Kale and Carrot Salad

(As seen in *Living with Crohn's and Colitis* by Dede Cummings and Jessica Black, N.D.)

Serves 2–4

Dressing
1 tablespoon sesame oil
1 tablespoon olive oil
⅓ cup brown rice vinegar
1 teaspoon pure maple syrup

Salad
5 large carrots, sliced
1 bunch kale, chopped
2 tablespoons sesame seeds
2 tablespoons hemp seeds

Dressing
Mix all ingredients.

Salad
Steam carrots and kale until soft but still crunchy and cool. Mix with seeds, coat with dressing mixture, and store in the refrigerator. Flavors will mix if left overnight. Serve chilled.

Easy Salmon Salad

(As seen in *Living with Crohn's and Colitis* by Dede Cummings and Jessica Black, N.D.)

Serves 2–4

2 (10 oz.) cans wild boneless, skinless salmon
½ cup mayonnaise, organic
½ cup minced carrots
½ cup minced apples
¼ cup sweet relish, organic and sweetened naturally

Mix all ingredients in a large bowl. Serve chilled with crackers, on a salad, or alone.

Sam's Chickpea Salad with Lemon and Parmesan

Serves 2

1 (12 oz.) can chickpeas, drained and rinsed
1 teaspoon fresh lemon juice or ½ teaspoon bottled lemon juice
1 tablespoon olive oil
Pinch of salt
¼ cup grated Parmigiano-Reggiano
Parsley, for garnish

Put all ingredients in a bowl, toss, and serve—delicious chilled and topped with fresh parsley.

> Chickpeas, or garbanzo beans, are terrific for their added fiber content, which is a real benefit for digestive support!

Sam's Butternut Squash Salad

Serves 4

1 fresh butternut squash (about 1 pound), peel the skin, and discard
   the seeds inside and chop into cubes
¼ cup raisins
¼ cup canola oil
1 tablespoon sherry vinegar
1 tablespoon fresh ginger, minced
Salt and freshly ground black pepper, to taste.

In a ceramic salad bowl, combine the squash, raisins, oil, vinegar,
and ginger and sprinkle with salt and pepper.

   Serve immediately, or store in the fridge and serve later. You can
also put a large dollop on a bed of fresh lettuce or spinach leaves.

Greens and Avocado Salad

Serves 4

4–5 cups baby salad greens
½–1 cup raw cashew pieces
¼ cup Caesar salad dressing (more or less to taste)
1 avocado, sliced

Toss greens together with cashew pieces and salad dressing in a large mixing bowl. Serve, garnished with avocado slices.

Fish & Seafood Entrées

Salmon Burgers

Serves 4

1 (7½ oz.) can salmon
1 egg, slightly beaten
¼ cup onion, finely chopped
¼ cup salsa
¾ cup fresh bread crumbs

Drain salmon thoroughly, squeezing out excess moisture. In a bowl, flake salmon with a fork. Add egg, onion, salsa, and bread crumbs. Blend thoroughly until mixture is almost smooth.

Divide and form mixture into four patties. Place on spray-coated or oiled preheated grill or broiler pan. Place about 4 to 5 inches from heat and grill about 4 to 5 minutes per side.

Warm Salmon Salad and Crispy Potatoes

Serves 4

2 tablespoons extra virgin olive oil, divided
2 small yellow-fleshed potatoes, scrubbed and cut into ⅛-inch slices
½ teaspoon salt, divided
1 medium shallot, thinly sliced
2 teaspoons rice vinegar
¼ cup buttermilk
2 (7 oz.) cans boneless, skinless salmon, drained
4 cups arugula

Heat 1 tablespoon oil in a large nonstick skillet over medium-high heat. Add potatoes and cook, turning once, until brown and crispy, 5 to 6 minutes per side. Transfer to a plate and season with ¼ teaspoon salt; cover with foil to keep warm. Combine the remaining 1 tablespoon oil, ¼ teaspoon salt, shallot and vinegar in a small saucepan. Bring to a boil over medium heat. Remove from heat and whisk in buttermilk. Place salmon in a medium bowl and toss with the warm dressing. Divide arugula among four plates and top with the potatoes and salmon.

Lemon Steamed Fish

Serves 2

½ pound cod, halibut, scrod fillets or other mild white fish
2 tablespoons finely chopped onion
2 tablespoons finely chopped fresh parsley
½ teaspoon dill weed
⅛ teaspoon paprika
Dash of pepper
1 teaspoon lemon juice

Preheat oven to 375°F.

Center each fillet on a 12-inch square of foil. Sprinkle with onion, parsley, dill weed, paprika, pepper, and lemon juice. Fold foil over fillet to make a packet; pleat seams to securely enclose the packet and place on cookie sheet.

Bake for 30 minutes.

Recipe will serve 16 in a demonstration setting. This recipe is easy to prepare with little clean-up. It is also low in fat and carbohydrates.

Almond Crusted Fish

Serves 2

½ pound mild white fish fillets (sole, flounder, orange roughy, etc.)
⅙ cup sliced almonds
1 tablespoon reduced-fat margarine, melted
1 tablespoon lemon or lime juice
½ teaspoon Worcestershire sauce, low-sodium
¼ teaspoon paprika
⅛ teaspoon pepper
Nonstick spray

Preheat oven to 375°F. Coat pan with cooking spray. Rinse and pat fish dry, arrange in pan in a single layer.

In a small bowl, mix almonds, margarine, lemon or lime juice, Worcestershire sauce, paprika, and pepper. Top fillets with above mixture, spreading evenly.

Bake 12–15 minutes or until fish flakes easily.

Cracked Crab with Curry and Ginger Sauce

Serves 2

1 live crab
2 tablespoons olive oil
1 clove minced garlic
1 teaspoon minced ginger
1 teaspoon chopped scallions
1 tablespoon green pepper (optional)
1 heaping tablespoon curry power
½ teaspoon salt
1 teaspoon sugar
3 tablespoons dry white sauterne
½ cup chicken broth or water
1 tablespoon cornstarch (with 2 tablespoons warm water)

To prepare live crab
Drop in boiling water for two minutes. Remove immediately and plunge into cold water. Separate body and claws. Discard yellowish liquid and any undesirable parts of the crab. Chop crab, still in shell, using cleaver or sharp knife.

Sauce
Place wok (or skillet) over high heat; add oil.

When oil is very hot, add minced garlic, ginger, scallions (and optional peppers); stir fry for 30 seconds.

Add crab-in-shell and stir fry for 1 minute. Combine curry, sugar and salt with sauterne, and pour over crab. Stir fry 30 seconds, and then add broth (or water). Cook for 5 minutes and then add cornstarch mix; stir until thick.

Make sure not to overcook crab or it will toughen. Ignore the directions for preparing live crab if using pre-cracked, cooked crab. Double recipe for two or more, accordingly.

Poached or Steamed Lobster

Serves 4

4 live lobsters, about 1½ pounds each
2 cups water
1 bay leaf
6 peppercorns
Beurre blanc (see recipe page 68)
Salt, to taste

Put lobsters and the remaining ingredients, except the beurre blanc, in a large kettle with a tight-fitting cover. Cover closely and bring to a boil. Cook over high heat for about 10 minutes.

Split the lobsters in half and serve with the beurre blanc spooned over each half.

Beurre Blanc

(For Poached or Steamed Lobster, see page 67)

Makes 1 cup

2 tablespoons finely chopped shallots
½ cup dry white wine
1 teaspoon white wine vinegar
½ pound butter, at room temperature but not too soft
Freshly ground pepper, to taste

In a heavy saucepan combine the shallots, wine, vinegar, and pepper to taste. Bring to a boil. Have a wire whisk ready and the butter close by.

Cook over high heat, stirring vigorously with the whisk. Add the butter, about a tablespoon at a time, always beating vigorously with the whisk. Do not at any time allow the sauce to boil.

When all the butter is added, continue beating rapidly while removing the saucepan from the heat. Place it on a cool surface. The sauce should not be chilled but if it is excessively hot, it will separate.

Until the sauce is served, continue to stir at intervals to prevent curdling. If the sauce is not to be used immediately, let it stand in the warm saucepan, stirring occasionally but do not re-heat it.

Steve's Fish

Serves 2

1½ pounds wild, fresh-caught Pollock
½ cup dry white wine
3 small tomatoes
1 small onion
12 black Tuscan olives with pits
1 teaspoon olive oil or canola margarine
Parmesan cheese, to taste

Preheat oven to 350°F.

Wash and dry fish and place in a glass baking dish (1½ pounds of fish is good for 3 people). Pour white wine over the fish.

Cut up tomatoes in chunks and onions in half-moon slices and arrange over the top of the fish. Add black olives here and there. Add olive oil to sprinkle over the top.

Cover with aluminum foil and bake for 20 minutes. Then check the fish to see if it is done by flaking it with a fork, and bake, uncovered, a bit more. Before serving, sprinkle some freshly grated Parmesan cheese over the top.

This recipe works well with a tossed salad of romaine lettuce, red peppers sliced thin, sliced carrots, and avocado. A side dish of steamed rice is also perfect with this delicious and savory fish recipe that my husband makes for our happy household (see my Steamed Rice recipe on page 108).

Wild Rice & Crabmeat Dish

Serves 2–4

2 cups wild rice, cooked
1 cup basmati white rice, cooked
1 cup crabmeat
1½ cups celery, chopped
1 green pepper, chopped
1 medium onion
1 cup pimento
1 cup shrimp, divided

Sauce
1 pound mushrooms
1 tablespoon butter
3 cups mushroom soup, divided

Preheat oven to 325°F.

Combine wild rice, rice, crabmeat, celery, green pepper, onion, and pimento. Add 1½ cans of mushroom soup and ½ cup of shrimp. Place mixture in baking dish and bake for 1½ hours.

Sauce
Brown mushrooms in butter. Add remaining 1½ cans of mushroom soup and remaining ½ cup shrimp. Heat to a low boil. Pour hot mushroom sauce over rice mixture and serve.

Baked Scallops

Serves 4

1 pound fresh scallops
½ cup half-and-half
½ cup white wine
2 tablespoons butter
1 cup seasoned breadcrumbs

Preheat oven to 375°F. Cover scallops with half-and-half in a greased casserole dish. Add a splash of white wine. Dab with pats of butter. Sprinkle liberally with seasoned breadcrumbs. Cover and bake for 45 minutes.

Bobbie Klaw's Fish Curry

Serves 4

2 tablespoons butter
3 onions, chopped
2 cloves garlic
3 tablespoons parsley, chopped
1½ teaspoons turmeric
1 teaspoon salt
1½ tablespoons coconut
1½ teaspoon curry
3 tomatoes, cut into wedges
3 tablespoons yogurt
1½ pounds scrod, cut into small pieces

Heat oil, sauté onions, garlic, and parsley until onions are lightly browned. Add turmeric, salt, coconut, and curry. Mix well. Cook for 3 minutes.

Add tomatoes and cook for 10 minutes. Stir in yogurt and cook for 5 minutes over medium heat. Add fish, cover well with sauce and let curry come to a boil.

Cover and simmer for 10 minutes.

Broiled Marinated Fish

Serves 4

2–4 pounds fish
2 teaspoons powdered cumin
1 clove garlic, crushed
Juice of ½ lemon
1 teaspoon dried savory, crushed
1 cup soy sauce
1 tablespoon olive oil

Rinse fish and pat dry. Cut in 3 diagonal slashes about 1½ inch apart with a sharp, thin-bladed knife. Place fish in a shallow baking dish and combine all remaining ingredients.

Pour mixture over the fish on each side and marinate in the refrigerator for 4 hours.

Preheat broiler for 10 minutes. Remove fish from marinade and lightly pat dry.

Broil 10 minutes on each side, basting twice with marinade.

Crab-Stuffed Flounder

Serves 4

4 tablespoons butter or margarine, divided
1 small onion, chopped
¼ cup celery, chopped
¼ cup sweet red pepper, chopped
¼ pound crabmeat, picked over and flaked
½ cup soft breadcrumbs
3 teaspoons lemon juice, divided
½ teaspoon salt
⅛ teaspoon pepper
Few drops liquid red pepper seasoning
4 small flounder fillets (about 4 ounces each)
Paprika, to taste
Lemon wedges, for garnish
Parsley, for garnish

Preheat oven to 350°F. Butter small shallow baking dish.

Sauté onion, celery, and red pepper in 2 tablespoons butter in saucepan until soft (about 2 minutes). Mix in crabmeat, breadcrumbs, 1 teaspoon lemon juice, salt, pepper, and red pepper seasoning.

Place flounder fillets skin side up in saucepan. Mound crab mixture in center of fillets. Overlap ends of fillets over top of stuffing. Fasten with wooden picks. Place in prepared dish.

Melt remaining 2 tablespoons butter in small saucepan; stir in lemon juice. Pour over fish and sprinkle with paprika. Bake in oven for 18–20 minutes or until fish flakes when pierced with a fork. Garnish with lemon wedges and parsley.

> This dish works well when served with herb-seasoned rice.

Catalan Seafood Stew from Barcelona, Catalonia, Spain

My son, Sam, lives in Barcelona, so he is learning a whole new culture and language (maybe 2 languages, with Catalan after mastering Castilian Spanish), not to mention he is a foodie who loves to cook. I love how he integrates food into his life, and uses it to explore a new culture and language. When we made this recipe, adapted from a few different recipes and what fresh fish was available at the central market in Barcelona, we learned a lot about the diversity of fish and the traditions of a wonderful culture. The use of a mortar and pestle is unusual where I live in Vermont, but in Catalonia, Spain, it is a kitchen necessity.

4 slices rap (monkfish)
4 slices dorada (sea bream)
4 slices cabracho (scorpion fish)
6 large prawns
12 mussels
2 tablespoons olive oil
1 clove garlic, minced
1 slice bread
1 Monkfish liver (this may be hard to find!)
1 cup toasted almonds
¼ teaspoon chili
1 tablespoon parsley
¼ teaspoon saffron
1 tablespoon sweet pepper, diced
1 tablespoon flour
2 cups fish stock, or water, or vegetable stock
1 pound potatoes, cut into slices, or cubes
A few drops of brandy
½ cup white wine
½ cup alioli (garlic mayonnaise)

(continued on next page)

Rinse and clean the fish and scrub the mussels well under running water, then put to one side. Heat the olive oil in a large pot, and fry the garlic and the bread slice. When the garlic and bread turn golden, remove and then fry the fish liver.

To make the picada, take fried bread into breadcrumbs, crumble between your fingers, and put in the mortar along with the fried garlic, fish liver, toasted almonds, chili, parsley, and saffron. Add the sweet pepper and flour to a little olive oil and place in the mortar. Grind all these ingredients into a paste, and then put the mashed ingredients into the pot. Heat on high and turn down to medium to simmer.

Add the water and the potatoes, and slowly cook on a low heat. When the potatoes are almost done, add all the fish, stir in the brandy and white wine and mix together with a spoon. Add the prawns and the (unopened) mussels; cover with a lid and cook for a further 15 minutes.

Add a bit of alioli to the stew to taste. Serve in ceramic bowls with a Spanish red table wine.

Connie's Grilled Salmon

Serves 4

1 pound wild salmon fillet
2 tablespoons olive oil (1 tablespoon for seasoning plus 1 tablespoon
   for ginger sauce)
Juice from 1 lemon (1 tablespoon for seasoning plus 1 tablespoon for
   ginger sauce)

Ginger sauce
1 tablespoon lemon juice
1 tablespoon olive oil
1 clove garlic, minced
2 tablespoons grated ginger
½ teaspoon soy sauce
2 tablespoons chopped cilantro
1 teaspoon dijon mustard
Salt and pepper, to taste

Season fillet with dash of lemon juice, pepper, and olive oil. Place
on pre-heated grill and cook salmon 6-8 minutes per side. Brush
on marinade and serve.

Serve with new red potatoes and tarragon butter (mix soft butter with
chopped tarragon).

Alex's Nori Wrapped Salmon

Not vegan, not raw, but delicious!

1 tablespoon olive oil
1 tablespoon pommery mustard (the whole mustard grain is kept
  intact and it's delicious!)
¼ teaspoon wasabi powder (I always use more because I like mine
  spicy)
2 (8oz.) salmon filets
1 sheet nori
Salt and pepper, to taste

Pre-heat oven to 450°F.

Mix olive oil, salt, and pepper. Rub salmon with mixture.

Mix mustard and wasabi (I use a dash of olive oil here as well).
Spread mixture on the sheet of nori.

Place the salmon fillet in the middle of the nori sheet and wrap
it up as you would a present so the the fish is covered completely
(sometimes the nori crinkles and cracks, so I moisten it with olive
oil to smooth it out).

Place the wrapped fish in a lightly oiled baking dish. Bake for
10 minutes per inch of thickness, being careful not to overcook.

The nori keeps the salmon moist and tender. Therefore, you can skin the
fillets before you wrap them. Place a fillet skin-side down on a cutting
board. Press on top of the filet using your whole hand. Insert the blade
of a sharp knife between the meat and the skin and, applying steady
pressure, slice the skin off using steady strokes.

You can mix any of your favorite herbs with the olive oil, salt, and
pepper.

You can prepare as many "parcels" as you'd like. They are also great the
next day, chilled.

Sharon's Oven-Fried Fish

Serves 4

1 pound fresh cod, cut into about 2-inch pieces
1 egg (or two egg whites if you're concerned about fat/cholesterol),
   beaten well
1 bag good-quality potato chips (I use vinegar and salt), processed
   into fine crumbs

Dip cod pieces into the egg. Coat with potato chip crumbs.

Bake on a cookie sheet for 7–10 minutes at 400°F. (I line mine
with nonstick foil or you could use parchment paper.)

So simple, so good! No added oil necessary—the oil from the chips is
all you need to cook it.

Meat, Poultry, & Vegetarian Entrées

Excellent Savory Tofu Stew

Serves 6–8

¼ cup olive or vegetable oil
3 onions, thinly sliced
4 carrots, thinly sliced
4–5 stalks celery, thinly sliced
2–3 cloves garlic, minced or pressed
1 cup firm tofu (press out excess water)
1½ cups zucchini or yellow squash, ¼-inch slices
2 fresh tomatoes, diced
1 tablespoon dried basil
2 bay leaves
2 cups tomato juice
⅓ cup soy sauce (or tamari)

Heat oil in a large lidded pot over medium heat. Add onion, carrots, celery, and garlic, cooking until onions are transparent. Add tofu, zucchini or squash, and tomatoes. Simmer a bit, and then add spices. Simmer for 2–3 minutes. Pour in tomato juice and soy sauce; stir.

Reduce heat to low, cover pot, and simmer for one hour.

Tofu is a soy-based, protein-rich food made by coagulating soy milk with resulting curds pressed into soft white blocks.

Eggplant and Walnuts with Cardamom

Serves 2–4

4 tablespoons olive oil, divided
2 teaspoons garlic, minced
1 medium onion, chopped
½ pound mushrooms, sliced
1¼ pound eggplant, peeled and diced
2 teaspoons curry powder
½ teaspoon ground cardamom
3 large tomatoes, peeled and diced (or 1½ cups canned)
2 tablespoons lemon juice
4 tablespoons parsley
¾ cup walnuts, chopped
Pinch salt

Heat 1 tablespoon of oil in a heavy pot. Add garlic and onions; sauté until soft. Stir in mushrooms and simmer, covered, for 3–4 minutes. Add eggplant, curry, and cardamom. Cook over medium-low heat, covered, for 5–10 minutes (or until cooked through). Stir once and then stir in tomatoes and heat through. Add lemon juice, remaining oil, parsley, walnuts, and a pinch of salt; heat through.

Serve hot or cold over rice or noodles.

Cardamom is a very exotic spice, unique and really good. It should be bought ground (powdered), not whole.

Steve's Chicken-Marango

Serves 4

1 chicken (2–3 pounds), cut
2 tablespoons olive oil
1 clove garlic, minced
5 green onions (scallions), minced
½ cup white wine
¼ teaspoon thyme
¼ cup tomato sauce
1 tablespoon parsley
Salt and pepper, to taste

In a large heavy skillet, brown chicken in olive oil until golden. Remove pieces to a warm bowl; salt and pepper. Add onions and garlic to skillet; heat until transparent and golden.

Add wine, thyme, and tomato sauce to skillet, scraping bottom; heat until bubbly.

Add chicken; cover and cook at 350°F for 30 minutes on stove.

Lea's Okra Lamb Stew

Serves 4

1 pound lamb stew meat
2 large onions, sliced
1 pound tender okra
1 tomato, cut
½ cup tomato sauce
Juice of 1 lemon
Salt and pepper, to taste

Braise meat until brown. Add onions and cook until soft.

Wash okra, peel tips and keep in bowl of cold water as you clean the tips; drain off water and add to meat mixture. Add to remaining ingredients and cook until okra is tender, about 30–40 minutes.

Turmeric Lentils with Spinach or Chard

(As seen in *Living with Crohn's and Colitis* by Dede Cummings and Jessica Black, N.D.)

Serves 4

2 cups red lentils
4 cups water
1 vegetable bouillon cube, no-salt-added
2 tablespoons olive oil
1 tablespoon mustard seeds
1 onion
2 cloves garlic, minced
1 tablespoon butter
2 teaspoons turmeric
½ teaspoon cumin
1 teaspoon coriander
1 bunch chard, chopped or 1 large bunch spinach, chopped
½ head Napa cabbage (optional)
1 pound seasoned chicken sausage, cooked (optional)
Sea salt, to taste

In saucepan, add lentils, water, and bullion and bring to boil, covered. Reduce heat to medium low and continue to simmer until all water has been absorbed. This will usually take a little while, so be patient. If all water is absorbed and lentils are not soft, keep adding more water until lentils are soft.

In a separate large saucepan or soup pot, heat olive oil on medium low heat and add mustard seeds for about 1 minute. Make sure to cover with a lid because mustard seeds begin to jump once they are hot. Add onion, garlic, and butter and sauté until soft. Add all spices while stirring and then add chard and the cabbage and chicken sausage, if you are including them. Once vegetables are cooked slightly but still crunchy, add lentils and cook a little longer until flavors have mingled. Add sea salt to taste and serve over brown rice or quinoa.

Mushroom Risotto with Cashews and Parmesan

(As seen in *Living with Crohn's and Colitis* by Dede Cummings and Jessica Black, N.D.)

This recipe takes some time to prepare but is definitely worth it! Take the time and you and your guests will be pleasantly impressed.

Serves 4

1 teaspoon butter
2 tablespoons olive oil, divided
3 cloves garlic
1½ pounds fresh, wild mushrooms of various kinds (procini, morels, shiitake, Portobello), cleaned, trimmed, and cut into thin strips
1 medium yellow onion, chopped
6–7 cups vegetable or chicken broth
1½ cups Arborio rice
⅓ cup Marsala wine
⅔ cup dry white wine
⅓ cup Parmesan cheese, grated (optional)
½ cup ground cashews
½ cup chopped flat-leaf parsley
Sea salt, to taste

Heat the butter and 1 tablespoon of olive oil in a large saucepan over medium heat. Sauté garlic for one minute. Add the mushrooms and sea salt and sauté until the mushrooms release their moisture, get tender, and begin to color around the edges. Heat the remaining tablespoon of olive oil in another saucepan over medium heat and sauté the onion until it is soft and barely golden. At the same time, heat the broth in a soup pan over low heat and keep it warm.

   Add the rice to the sautéed onion pan and stir together for a few minutes. Add the Marsala and keep stirring as it reduces, or

(continued on next page)

cooks away. Add the white wine and after it has reduced, stir in the sautéed mushrooms and about one cup of the hot broth. Adjust the temperature to a low medium so that the broth simmers gently with the rice and stir slowly as it reduces. When more than half of the broth has reduced, add another cup of the broth while stirring in the same manner. Continue this process until most of the broth is used and the rice is al dente. This will take about 20–25 minutes. When the rice has reached the right texture, stir in the last cup of broth, Parmesan cheese, and ground cashews and prepare for serving. Right before serving, add the chopped parsley.

Easy Marinade for Chicken, Salmon, or Tofu

(As seen in *Living with Crohn's and Colitis* by Dede Cummings and Jessica Black, N.D.)

Serves 4

1 cup wheat-free tamari
½ cup honey
½ cup dark sesame oil
1 tablespoon grated ginger
1 clove minced garlic

Mix all ingredients together. Coat salmon, chicken, or tofu and allow to sit overnight before preparing.

Coconut Brown Rice

(As seen in *Living with Crohn's and Colitis* by Dede Cummings and Jessica Black, N.D.)

2 cups brown rice
4 cups filtered water
2–3 tablespoons creamed coconut
½ teaspoon pure maple syrup

Bring rice and water to a boil in a saucepan. Allow to boil for 2 minutes, reduce heat to low. Then add coconut and maple syrup, cover, and allow to simmer for 15 minutes. Remove from heat and keep covered for another 5 minutes. Serve warm with your favorite vegetable dish.

Wild Rice Casserole

Serves 4

1 cup wild rice
1 onion, chopped
3 celery stalks
1 teaspoon salt
½ cup white wine
2 tablespoons butter
1 quart broth

Preheat oven to 325°F. Combine all ingredients. Place in casserole.
Bake covered for 2 hours. This dish freezes well.

Christie's Thai Chicken with Basil

Serves 4

1 pound chicken breast, cut into cubes
2 tablespoons vegetable oil, divided
1 teaspoon chili paste (substitute dried red chili pepper and 2
    tablespoons minced garlic)
¾ cup straw mushrooms
½ cup baby corn
3 tablespoons fish sauce
1 tablespoon sugar
1 cup fresh basil leaves (if available, use holy basil)

Cut the chicken into cubes. Heat a wok, add 1 tablespoon oil. Add
the chili paste and fry on moderate heat, stirring until fragrant (3
minutes). Add remaining 1 tablespoon of oil. Turn heat to high.
Add chicken breast and stir-fry until cooked throughout.

Add the mushrooms and baby corn to the wok. Mix well.
Add the fish sauce, sugar, and basil leaves. Stir until the sugar has
dissolved and the basil. Serve over rice.

Molly's Rancho Bean Casserole

Serves 4

1 pound dried pinto beans
3 tablespoons margarine
1½ cups onions, thinly sliced
2 cloves garlic, crushed
1 cup dried green pepper
1 tablespoon chili powder
1 can (2 pounds and 3 ounces) tomatoes
½ cup maple syrup
Mustard, to taste
Salt and pepper, to taste

Wash beans, cover with cold water and soak overnight. Drain beans, add fresh water, cover and bring to a slow boil. Simmer over low heat for 1 hour or until beans are tender. Drain and save 1 cup liquid. Sauté onions in margarine, green peppers, and garlic for 5 minutes.

Add chili powder, tomatoes, maple syrup, salt, pepper, and mustard. Mix well.

Stir tomato mixture into beans and heat up at 350°F.

Julie's Rice Dish

My friend, food writer, Julie Potter, wrote, "This is something my mom would make when we were kids. I mostly remember the cheesy comfortableness." The vegetables give it a nice crunch.

Serves 4

4 cups water
2 cups white or brown rice
1 tablespoon butter
½ large onion
3 ribs celery
3 carrots, peeled
½ red pepper, diced
½ teaspoon dried thyme
1 teaspoon dried basil
1½ -2 teaspoons dried oregano
2–3 ripe tomatoes, chopped
4 ounces cheddar cheese, cubed
Salt and pepper, to taste

Bring water to a boil. Add rice, cover, lower heat to simmer, and cook until just tender.

While rice is cooking, melt butter in a large skillet over medium heat. Add onion, celery, and carrots, all cut to a similar dice. Sauté over medium heat, taking care not to brown until just starting to turn translucent. Add red pepper and continue to sauté until veggies are cooked, but still crisp. Season with salt and pepper, and add thyme, basil, and oregano. Add cooked rice and ripe tomatoes. Combine ingredients gently and top evenly with cheddar cheese. Lower heat and cover pan until cheese is just melted. Serve.

Julie's Pistou

Another childhood favorite of my friend, Julie Potter's, who grew up on a farm in Southern Vermont. This was always a late summer or early harvest meal based on what was in the garden.

Serves 4

1 tablespoon butter
1 medium onion, diced
1 leek, diced
2 large tomatoes, peeled, seeded, and crushed
4 cups chicken or vegetarian stock or water
½ pound fresh green beans
3 potatoes, cut into bite-sized pieces
Approximately ¼ pound spaghetti, broken in half
2 cloves garlic, crushed
Several basil leaves, crushed
2 tablespoons olive oil
2–3 tablespoons broth (chicken or vegetarian)
4 tablespoons Parmesan cheese, grated
Salt and pepper, to taste

In a medium heavy pot over med low heat, melt butter and slowly cook onion and leek. Add tomatoes. Add stock or water to pot and bring to a boil. Add fresh green beans and potatoes. Season with salt and pepper. When veggies are almost cooked (about 15 minutes) add spaghetti. Reduce heat and finish cooking very slowly.

While cooking, pound garlic with several basil leaves. Add, still pounding, olive oil and 2–3 tablespoons chicken or vegetarian broth. Serve soup, dividing pesto and Parmesan cheese between portions.

White beans, zucchini, and carrots can all be added, and if you are in a hurry, cheat and use already prepared basil pesto.

Vegetarian Stuffed Peppers

Serves 4

½ cup rice
½ pound mushrooms
2 tablespoons butter
½ cup chopped blanched almonds
2 tablespoons flour
½ cup thin cream
1½ teaspoons salt

Preheat oven to 350°F. Cook rice according to Dede's basic rice directions (see page 108), white or brown. Sauté mushrooms in butter. Sauté almonds separately. Sprinkle flour on mushrooms. Add cream, stirring until it thickens. Once the cream mix has thickened, take a soup spoon and carefully spoon the mixture into the pepper cavity, spoonful by spoonful, until full. When finished, try to find the right top and place it on the finished pepper base, and arrange in a baking dish that has a bit of oil on the bottom.

Bake for ½-1 hour.

Chicken Tarragon

Serves 6

2 chickens (2½ pounds each), cut into pieces
2 tablespoons olive oil
1 cup dry vermouth
2 tablespoons fresh tarragon leaves
Salt and pepper, to taste

Brown chicken in oil in large heavy pot over high heat. Reduce heat, add vermouth, tarragon, salt, and pepper. Turn chicken in sauce. Cover pot, cook over low heat for 45 minutes.

Serve with rice.

Roasted Vegetables

Serves 8–10

1 pound small potatoes, cut in ¾-inch dice
1 large (about 1 pound) celery root, peeled and cut in ¾-inch dice
4 medium parsnips (about 1 pound) peeled and cut in ¾-inch dice
4 medium carrots (about 1 pound) peeled and cut in ¾-inch dice
4 shallots, peeled and quartered
2 red bell peppers, seeded and cut in ¾-inch dice
5 tablespoons olive oil
2 teaspoons kosher salt
½ teaspoon freshly ground pepper
4 cloves garlic, minced
2 tablespoons chopped rosemary or thyme leaves, or a combination

Preheat oven to 425°F.

In a large bowl, combine potatoes, celery root, parsnips, carrots, shallots, bell peppers, olive oil, salt, and pepper. Toss. Spread over vegetables in a single layer over sheet pans and roast, stirring often, until tender and well-browned (about 40–45 minutes). Sprinkle with the garlic and herbs. Toss and roast for 2 minutes.

Remove from oven and serve.

Stuffed Eggplant Creole

Serves 2–4

1 small eggplant
5–6 mushrooms, chopped
3 large cloves garlic
¼ cup onion, chopped
¼ cup pepper, chopped
2 cups drained canned tomatoes
¼ cup celery
⅓ cup breadcrumbs
½ cup cheese, grated
Salt and pepper, to taste

Preheat oven to 350°F.

Cut eggplant into halves, scoop out pulp, and chop it. Leave a shell ¼-inch thick.

Sauté mushrooms. In a separate skillet, Mince garlic, onion, and pepper and heat. Add eggplant pulp, tomatoes, and celery. Simmer until eggplant is tender. Mix in breadcrumbs, salt, and pepper. Add sautéed mushrooms. Fill eggplant shells with mixture and grated cheese. Bake in a pan with a little water until thoroughly heated, about 15 minutes).

Sam's Butternut Squash and Hazelnut Lasagna

This recipe was adapted from *Gourmet* magazine via the website www.epicurious.com.

Serves 6

Squash filling
1 large onion, chopped
3 tablespoons butter
3 pounds butternut squash, peeled, seeded, and cut into ½-inch pieces
1 tablespoon garlic, minced
1 teaspoon salt
¼ teaspoon white pepper
2 tablespoons chopped fresh Italian (flat-leaf) parsley
4 teaspoons chopped fresh sage
½ cup chopped pine nuts

Sauce
1 teaspoon garlic, minced
3 tablespoons butter
5 tablespoons spelt flour
5 cups low-fat milk (see substitution chart on page 159 if needed)
1 bay leaf
1 teaspoon salt
¼ teaspoon white pepper

Assembling lasagna
12 (7- x 3½-inch) sheets soy or brown rice lasagna (½ pound)
½ pound fresh mozzarella, coarsely grated (2 cups)
1 cup finely grated Parmigiano-Reggiano (3 ounces)

Squash filling
Cook the onion in butter in a deep 14-inch cast-iron skillet over medium heat, stirring until onion is golden. Add squash, garlic, salt,

and white pepper. Cook, stirring occasionally, until squash is fork-tender. Mix in parsley, sage, and nuts. Set aside and cool.

Sauce

Cook garlic in butter in a 3-quart heavy saucepan over moderately low heat, stirring, 1 minute. Whisk in flour and cook *roux*, whisking, 3 minutes. Add milk in a stream, whisking. Add bay leaf and bring to a boil, whisking constantly, then reduce heat and simmer, whisking occasionally, 10 minutes. Whisk in salt and white pepper and remove from heat. Discard bay leaf. (Cover surface of sauce with wax paper if not using immediately.)

Assembling lasagna

Cook lasagna noodles in large pasta pot until al dente and rinse with cold water to stop cooking and set aside for assembly.

Preheat oven to 425°F.

Toss cheeses together. Spread ½ cup sauce in an oiled 13- x 9- x 2-inch glass baking dish, and cover with three pasta sheets, arranged with a bit of space between.

Spread with 1 cup sauce and one third of the filling, then sprinkle with a heaping cup of cheese. Repeat, layering 2 more times, beginning with pasta and ending with cheese. Top with remaining pasta sheets, remaining sauce, and remaining cheese.

Cover the baking dish with foil and bake for 30 minutes. Remove foil, sprinkle with any extra cheese, and bake until golden and bubbling, about 10 to 15 minutes more. Let lasagna stand 15 to 20 minutes before cutting and serving.

> Filling and sauce can be made 1 day ahead and kept separately, covered, and chilled. Bring to room temperature before assembling.

Sam's Asparagus-Parmesan Risotto

This recipe was adapted from *Gourmet* magazine via the website www.epicurious.com.

Serves 3–4

1 pound asparagus (break off the bottoms with your hands), cut into
   1-inch pieces, tips reserved
4–6 cups chicken or vegetable stock
2 tablespoons olive oil
3 tablespoons butter, divide in half
1 medium red onion, diced
1½ cups Arborio rice
½ cup dry white wine
½ cup Parmesan cheese, freshly grated
Salt, to taste

Steam about half the asparagus stalks and cook until quite soft, at least 5 minutes. Rinse quickly under cold water to stop the cooking, and set aside.

In a blender or food processor, add the cooked asparagus with just enough water to puree until smooth; set aside.

Add vegetable or chicken stock in a medium saucepan and heat over low heat. Measure oil and 1 tablespoon butter in a large (at least 12 inches), cast-iron skillet over medium heat, until bubbling; then add the onion, stirring occasionally until it softens, which takes approximately 5 minutes.

Add rice and cook, stirring occasionally, until it is pearl-colored which takes about 2 to 3 minutes. Add white wine and let liquid evaporate until almost gone. Add a bit of salt to taste. Next, slowly add the heated stock, stirring occasionally. Each time stock evaporates, add more. After 15 minutes or so, add remaining asparagus pieces and tips, continuing to add stock as needed. In

5 minutes, begin tasting the rice to make sure it is tender, but not too crunchy—this may take around 30 minutes. When it finally is the right consistency, add ½ cup asparagus puree. Remove the pan from heat and add remaining butter. Then add Parmesan and stir, adjusting seasoning as desired. Risotto should be slightly soupy. Serve immediately with a tossed salad (see Lynne's Summer Salad on page 132).

Suzanne's Hippy Yum Yum Steamed

This dish might not look very pretty, but it tastes great and is very easy to digest!

Serves 4

2 cups brown rice, any kind
3½ cups water
1 cup cut fresh kale leaves
2 cups fresh spinach leaves
1 cup fresh broccoli
2 carrots, peeled
1 red pepper sliced (optional)
1 zucchini, sliced (optional)
1½ cups chick peas (fresh and cooked or canned)
¾ cup hummus (see page 116)
Bragg® liquid aminos, to taste
Grated fresh Parmesan cheese, about a half a cup or more to taste
   (optional if sensitive to dairy)

Boil water for brown rice and simmer while cooking. When rice has a half an hour left, steam veggies and chick peas in any kind of steamer. When veggies have steamed for half an hour, sprinkle on Parmesan cheese, if using. When veggies look a little more cooked than al dente (usually up to 15 minutes), turn down to a simmer. When rice is done, dump rice in big bowl, dump veggies and chick peas on top, mix with hummus and liquid aminos.

Hippy Yum Yum Salad

This dish looks funny but tastes great!

Serves 4

1 red onion
⅓ cup chives
1 medium-sized red potato
½ large sweet potato
⅓ cup olive oil
Pinch of fresh rosemary
2 medium heads of romaine lettuce
2 shredded, sliced or peeled carrots
1 avocado
½ cup hummus (see page 116)
⅓ cup balsamic vinegar
Pinch of fresh dill
Juice of half a lemon

Cut up onion, chives, and two potatoes (very thinly sliced). Dump olive oil in large frying pan. Put in onion, potato, chives, and rosemary into frying pan. Stir occasionally.

Cut up romaine lettuce, carrots, and avocado into bowl. When frying pan ingredients have browned and are sizzling, dump them in with the salad, pour in balsamic, mix with hummus and lemon juice and sprinkle with dill.

> Salmon, sardines, chicken, or chickpeas can be added for protein.

Connie's Grilled Veggies and Turkey Burgers

Serves 4–6

Marinade
¼ cup olive oil
Juice of one lemon
Splash of balsamic vinegar
A few shakes of pepper

Veggies
1 zucchini, sliced lengthwise, ¼-inch thick
2 red, green, orange, or yellow peppers, sliced
¾ red onion, thickly sliced
1 bunch asparagus, sliced
7–8 mushrooms, sliced (optional)

Turkey burgers
2½ pounds lean, ground turkey
1 pound crumbled gorgonzola
⅓ cup red onion
3 cloves garlic

Bread
1 pound pan rustique, or all-natural flatbread

Turkey burgers
Mix patties and set aside.

Veggies
Put vegetables all in a zip-lock bag with marinade and shake it up, then refrigerate for at least one hour

Arrange vegetables on preheated grill and grill on moderate heat, covering the grill for first 5–10 minutes.

Start to turn vegetables over and repeat as necessary (black grill lines are one indication of doneness).

When vegetables are almost done, put the burgers on and cook next to vegetables.

Bread
Slice bread thickly and brush inside with olive oil.

Towards the end of cooking, add the bread slices to the edges of the grill and heat up both sides.

Serve on platters family-style.

Serve with Steve's Rawsome Guacamole (see page 112) as an appetizer with carrots.

As a variation, try Greek Burgers using locally-raised ground lamb mixed with feta (instead of the gorgonzola) and add one clove of garlic, and two tablespoons of fresh chopped mint. For a burger topping, mix ½ cup Greek yogurt, two tablespoons of chopped, fresh, mint, and ¼ cup of chopped Greek olives.

Alex's Raw Tacos

Serves 4

Small romaine lettuce leaves
1 (16 oz.) jar mango or tomato salsa (store-bought can be used if fresh
  and organic)
1 cup walnuts
1–2 tablespoons soy sauce or shoyu
Homemade Steve's Rawsome Guacamole (see page 112) or 1 (16 oz.)
  jar store-bought organic guacamole
1 cup raw cashews

Cover the cashews with an inch of water and soak for 1–2 hours.

Wash and dry lettuce leaves. Set aside.

In a food processor, or Vitamix® blender, add walnuts and soy
sauce and pulse a few times so that the mixture resembles cooked
ground beef. Set aside.

Drain the cashews and transfer to blender. Add ½ cup water (or
almond milk) and blend until smooth and creamy.

Assembly
Take one lettuce leaf and spread guacamole on it. Layer some
walnut "meat," some fresh salsa, and a dollop of cashew cream.

Wrap it up and eat as many as you like! (They are actually very
filling.)

UJ's Chili (Bean Soup and Spicy Bean Dip)

Serves 4

3 sweet peppers (I usually use green, but you can use a red pepper
   for color)
3 tablespoons olive oil
1 yellow onion
3 green onions (scallions)
1 red onion
1 (10 oz.) can dark red kidney beans or black beans
¼ teaspoon dried chili pepper flakes (or to taste and tolerance for
   spice)
1 drop hot sauce, optional

Chop each pepper into tiny squares. In a medium-sized pot on
the stove, sauté the chopped peppers in olive oil for about 10–15
minutes (add a drop or two of hot sauce, and/or chili pepper flakes,
if desired).

Then chop the onions into little squares and add to pot. Cook
under a low flame for 10–15 minutes (add a drop or two of hot
sauce, if desired).

After the onions and peppers simmer awhile, add the beans.

Stir the contents while singing a Mexican-themed song. Reduce
heat to simmer for 1 hour to 1½ hours. Stir the pot every 20
minutes.

Some people in my family think this recipe tastes better when reheated
the next day. If there are any leftovers on day 3, you can put it in a
blender to make a spicy bean dip.

Side Dishes & Snacks

Brown Rice

I love this recipe and it is my staple for macrobiotic eating. Many people have trouble cooking brown rice and having it turn out decently, since it can be more temperamental than white rice. White rice, however, is a bit easier to digest, but if you cook brown rice this way, it, too, is easily digested and better for you than white rice. If you want to try this recipe for white rice, I like using basmati white rice.

There are also many different ways to prepare brown rice. Here's the most efficient way I found to cook brown rice on a stove. It takes about 35 minutes from when you start to when you're eating (which is pretty good for brown rice). This method works for both short-grain and long-grain brown rice, although I prefer long-grain. I've eaten hundreds of batches of brown rice using this method over the past 10 years.

I hope you find these recipes helpful. Brown rice became a staple of my diet after I studied macrobiotics during the mid-90s, and I eat it almost every week. I find it a great food for endurance activities and just general all-around wellbeing!

3 cups brown rice
Water
Salt, to taste
Tamari, wheat-free (for seasoning)

Put brown rice and water together in a pot with a lid. Use the ratio of 1½ cups water to 1 cup rice. (I normally make 3 cups rice with 4½ cups water for a single batch.)

Set the heat to maximum, and bring the rice/water to a boil, uncovered. Then put the lid on the pot, and reduce the heat to low-simmer. If your lid has a steam valve, keep it closed. Let the rice simmer for 20 minutes.

Turn off the heat, and let the rice sit in the covered pot for another 10 minutes (it's okay if you let the rice sit longer than 10 minutes, 20 or 30 minutes is fine too), but don't let it go any less. I prefer my rice to be slightly chewy, not mushy, so I usually remove the lid after 10 minutes. Be careful when you remove the lid, since a lot of steam may escape when you do.

After the rice is cooked, I normally scoop some into a bowl, and mix it with a little tamari and 1-2 tablespoons of sesame seeds. The sesame seeds add a lot of flavor to the rice. Sometimes I'll also eat it with steamed vegetables and blackened tempeh, both of which can be prepared while the rice is cooking.

You can store any leftover rice in a plastic container in the refrigerator and it will keep well for several days. Since I don't use a microwave, I usually just eat the leftovers cold. But when I'm not in the mood for cold rice, here's another tasty dish I make from the leftover rice:

In a small pot, add 1 teaspoon of oil (I prefer dark sesame oil because it adds a lot of flavor, but canola oil works well too), and heat it for about 1 minute on medium heat. Add some chopped vegetables (my favorites are onions, green onions, and bell peppers) to the pot, and sauté them in the oil for a few minutes. Once the vegetables are cooked, scoop in some of the leftover brown rice (I like to use 2 parts rice to 1 part vegetables). Mix it well with the vegetables. Reduce the heat slightly to medium-low, and cook the rice/vegetables for 3-4 minutes until the rice is hot, stirring about once every minute. Pour in a little tamari to taste, and mix it with the rice. Cook for another minute to sear in the flavor. Turn off the heat. Mix in 1-2 tablespoons sesame seeds. Eat and enjoy.

Steamed Veggies

Vegetables
Your choice of vegetables (such as broccoli, asparagus, string beans, kale, spinach, sugar snap peas, pea pods, or chard)

Ginger soy sauce
1 tablespoon fresh ginger
½ cup soy sauce
Rice vinegar or white wine vinegar, to taste

Vegetables
Clean and chop the vegetables to desired size and place in a steamer pot (or just in boiling water) until tender.

Serve with melted butter (for asparagus) or ginger soy sauce (particularly good when using string beans and pea pods).

Ginger soy sauce
Grate the fresh ginger into the soy sauce and add rice vinegar or white wine vinegar to taste (approximate ratio is 4 parts soy to 1 part vinegar).

If you want to try something different, try using fresh snap peas and sauté them in butter with a few cloves of diced garlic.

Easy and Quick Dried Beans

Serves 4

½ pound dry beans
½ tablespoon salt
Water, to cover

Preheat oven to 250°F.

Use a Dutch oven, put the beans inside, and sort through them to clean out anything.

Cover the beans by half with water and add some salt. Bring the pot to a boil.

After a rolling boil is reached, cover the pot and put it in the pre-heated oven.

After about 30 minutes, open the lid and check to make sure they are not drying out. Add more water as necessary, and check every 10–15 minutes thereafter.

In about an hour, the beans should be done—easy and cost-saving!

I always keep a few cans of organic refried low-fat black beans in my pantry. Also, a few cans of pinto beans are great to have in case you run out of time!

Dried beans need to be rinsed and soaked overnight in order to release gas and soften them for cooking. It is best to change the soaking water twice during the 8–12 hour period and remove any small stones. Cover the bottom of a pan with the beans and then fill with cold water. Lentils and split peas can be cooked directly and don't need to be soaked.

Steve Rawsome's Guacamole

Guacamole is one of my favorite foods, so I'd like to share my best guacamole recipe that I got from my friend, Steve. I tweak this recipe every time
I make it (thanks to my daughter, Emma).

    I went to my first raw potluck last night and brought a large batch of
this guacamole to share. I figured there would be leftovers, but by the end
of the night, the bowl was practically licked clean. People seemed to really
love it.

2 large avocados (or 3 small ones)
Juice of 2 limes (about ¼ cup)
1 medium tomato (or 2 Roma tomatoes), chopped
¾ cup chopped fresh cilantro
⅓ cup chopped green onion
1 teaspoon minced jalapeño pepper (red or green)
1 teaspoon sea salt

Put the avocado flesh into a bowl. Add the lime juice. Mash the
avocado and lime juice together with a fork until creamy.

    Fold in tomato, cilantro, green onion, jalapeño pepper, and
sea salt. Enjoy!

This guacamole works especially well as a dip for organic carrot and
celery sticks. It also goes well with flax crackers. If you aren't a raw
foodist, it goes well with tortilla chips, too.

Feel free to adjust the ingredient ratios to suit your tastes (i.e. more
green onion, more jalapeño, more or less salt, etc).

If you like spicy guacamole, feel free to double or triple the jalapeño (or
more). The version above is pretty mild.

Savory Squash

(As seen in *Living with Crohn's and Colitis* by Dede Cummings and Jessica Black, N.D.)

Serves 2

1 buttercup squash
2 tablespoons olive oil
¼ cup hemp or almond milk
2 tablespoons honey
Sea salt, to taste

Cut squash in half and scoop out seeds. Preheat oven to 400°F. Bake squash in baking pan, sliced side down in 2–3 inches of water for about an hour or until soft. Remove from the oven and allow to cool to handling temperature. Scoop meat out into saucepan and add remaining ingredients. Warm to serving temperature.

Red Lentil Dip

Serves 8–10

1 pound dried red lentils
6 cups water
16 cloves roasted garlic, peeled
1 tablespoon olive oil
4 teaspoons lemon juice
1½ tablespoons salt/pepper
2 tablespoons minced parsley

Boil lentils in water. Reduce heat to simmer. Cook, stirring until very soft (about 45 minutes). Drain through mesh sieve until thick, but not dry. Put in food processor until smooth. Add remaining ingredients except parsley. Process until smooth.

Serve with crackers and parsley garnish.

Teta's Aduki Bean Pate

Serves 4

1 cup dried aduki beans
1½ cup tahini
1 onion, finely chopped
4 cloves garlic, minced
1 bunch parsley, chopped
1 tablespoon fresh ginger, minced
1½ cups light-colored miso
Tamari, to taste (optional)

Cook aduki beans until very soft. Set aside.

Pour tahini into large frying pan and brown over medium heat. Stir in onion and fry for about 3 minutes. Turn off heat. Stir in garlic parsley, and fresh ginger. (All of these quantities can be adapted to taste once you know what you like.) Allow to sit together until cooled to room temperature.

In a large bowl, stir together aduki beans, tahini mix, and miso. Put through homogenizer or food processor to puree together. Add tamari if not salty enough. Garnish with parsley.

Serve with crudités or dry crackers or thicken (by using less water when cooking beans) to use as a sandwich spread, topped with lettuce and thin cucumber and red pepper slices.

Our Family Favorite (Sam's) Hummus

Serves 6–8

2 cups canned chickpeas
½ cup tahini (sesame seed paste)
¼ cup olive oil
2 cloves garlic, chopped
1 tablespoon ground cumin
1 tablespoon lemon juice
Salt and freshly ground black pepper, to taste
2 tablespoons fresh parsley, chopped (for garnish)

Put the chickpeas, tahini, oil, garlic, cumin, and lemon juice in a blender.

Add salt and pepper then, once blended, add some hot water as needed to help blend. Serve in a ceramic bowl with rice crackers and/or sliced carrots.

Garbanzo beans, or chickpeas, have a delicious, nutty taste—my family can eat a big bowl of this hummus with sliced carrots in a few minutes!

Chewy Granola Bars

Makes 4 dozen bars

3 cups quick oats
1 cup peanuts
1 cup raisins
1 cup shelled sunflower seeds
1½ teaspoon cinnamon
1 (14 oz.) can unsweetened condensed milk
½ cup butter (shortening), melted

Preheat oven to 325°F.

Line 15½- x 10½- x 1-inch pan with foil, and grease pan. Combine oats, peanuts, raisins, sunflower seeds, and cinnamon in large bowl. Add condensed milk and shortening. Toss until blended. Press into pan.

Bake for 30–40 minutes, let cool. Cut into bars and let cool. Remove from pan and peel off foil.

Yogurt Fruit Dip

Serves 12

2 cups plain fat-free yogurt
2 tablespoons brown sugar
1 tablespoon frozen orange juice concentrate, thawed
½ teaspoon vanilla extract
¼ teaspoon ground cinnamon

Line a strainer with a paper coffee filter or cheesecloth; place over bowl. Put yogurt in strainer; refrigerate for 8 hours. Discard liquid in bowl. Combine yogurt, brown sugar, orange juice concentrate, vanilla extract, and cinnamon; mix well. Serve with fresh fruit of your choice.

Cucumber-Dill Spread

Serves 9

1 (8 oz.) package fat-free cream cheese, softened
1 teaspoon lemon juice
1 teaspoon minced onion
¼ teaspoon dill weed
⅛ teaspoon salt
⅛ teaspoon black pepper
⅛ teaspoon prepared horseradish
Dash of hot pepper sauce
⅓ cup finely diced, peeled, and seeded cucumber

In a mixing bowl, beat cream cheese until smooth. Add remaining ingredients except cucumber. Blend until smooth. Fold in cucumber. Cover and chill for at least one hour.

Serve with fresh vegetables.

White Bean Dip

Serves 20

1 (15 oz.) can cannellini beans or great Northern beans, rinsed and
  drained
1 tablespoon lemon juice
2 tablespoons plain non-fat yogurt
2 tablespoons chopped fresh parsley
½ teaspoon freshly ground black pepper
¼ teaspoon hot pepper sauce
2 garlic cloves
Toasted pita bread or fresh vegetables

Place all ingredients in a food processor or blender, cover, and
process until smooth. Chill. Serve with toasted pita bread or
vegetables.

Oven-Fried Parmesan Chicken Strips

Serves 2

1 (6–8 oz.) boneless, skinless chicken breast, cut into strips (for faster cooking, try using a 6–8 ounce pack of lean chicken tenderloins)
¼ cup non-fat plain yogurt
¼ cup bread crumbs
1 tablespoon grated Parmesan cheese
½ tablespoon flour
¼ teaspoon paprika
Pinch of cayenne pepper
Nonstick spray

Preheat the oven to 450°F and spray cooking sheet. Place chicken strips in yogurt and refrigerate while preparing the rest of the ingredients.

In small bowl, mix the rest of the ingredients. Coat each piece of chicken with yogurt and dredge in crumb mixture, pressing down on both sides to get a coating of crumbs. Place chicken strips on cookie sheet. Bake for 15–20 minutes or until chicken is tender and juice run clear.

Apple Slaw

This is a fast and easy recipe that is crunchy and colorful.

Serves 8

1 small unpeeled red apple, diced
4 cups shredded cabbage
½ cup red onion, chopped
1 small green bell pepper, chopped
½ cup fat-free, light vanilla yogurt
2 tablespoons orange juice
1 tablespoon sucralose
Dash of cinnamon

Combine all ingredients in a medium-sized mixing bowl. Stir well. Refrigerate until ready to serve.

> Using pre-packaged cole slaw mix in place of the shredded cabbage reduces time. The cinnamon adds a nice taste, but may be left out.

Orange-Almond Salad

This is a light and refreshing salad that provides a good source of fiber.

Serves 4

3 cups assorted greens
2 navel oranges, peeled and separated into sections
½ cup thinly sliced celery
2 tablespoons chopped green onions
¼ cup cider vinegar
¼ cup sucralose
2 teaspoons olive or canola oil
¼ cup toasted slivered almonds

Combine greens, orange sections, celery, and green onions in a large bowl. Combine vinegar, sucralose, and oil in a small mixing bowl; stir until well blended, and drizzle over greens.

To serve, place greens on a serving plate and garnish with 1 tablespoon of almonds over each salad. Serve immediately.

> Sealed bags of salad greens may be used. Mandarin oranges may also be substituted for the navel oranges.

Four Bean Salad

Serves 8

1 (8 ½ oz.) can cut green beans, drained
1 (8 ½ oz.) can cut wax beans, drained
1 (8 ½ oz.) can lima beans, drained
1 (8 ½ oz.) can kidney beans, drained
½ cup thinly sliced red onion rings
½ cup chopped celery
¼ cup diced green pepper

Dressing
2 teaspoons Dijon mustard
2 tablespoons vinegar
½ teaspoon sugar
½ teaspoon dried thyme (or 1 teaspoon chopped fresh thyme)
½ teaspoon black pepper
1 clove garlic, crushed or minced
¼ cup olive oil

In a large mixing bowl, combine all the beans, onion, celery, and green pepper.

In a smaller mixing bowl whisk together the mustard, vinegar, sugar, thyme, pepper, and garlic. Whisking continually, add the oil in a slow, thin stream. Whisk until well blended. Pour the dressing over the bean mixture and toss to coat well. Cover and refrigerate 1–2 days before serving.

Carrot, Apple and Raisin Salad

Serves 8

1 large (8 oz.) apple, peeled and cored
2 teaspoons lemon juice
¾ pound raw carrots
3 tablespoons dark raisins
⅓ cup non-fat sour cream
3 tablespoons skim milk
1 or 2 packets sucralose
¼ teaspoon ground cinnamon
¼ teaspoon ground nutmeg

Peel, core, and shred apple. Place apple in large mixing bowl and toss with lemon juice. Peel and grate carrots. Toss carrots and raisins with apple.

Mix non-fat sour cream with milk, sweetener, cinnamon, and nutmeg in small bowl. Pour over carrot mixture, toss with rubber scraper to coat; divide into serving bowls.

Cover tightly with plastic wrap and chill for 1 hour or more.

For preparing in food processor

Fit food processor with metal chopping blade. Place non-fat sour cream, milk, lemon juice, sweetener, cinnamon, and nutmeg in bowl of food processor. Blend on and off to mix. Unplug food processor and remove metal chopping blade, leaving sour cream mixture in bottom of mixing bowl. Fit food processor with grating tool. Grate carrots and apples directly into sour cream mixture. Turn off food processor and remove grating tool. Turn mixture into serving bowl. Sprinkle raisins over top of mixture and toss to blend.

Cover tightly with plastic wrap. Chill 1 hour or more before serving.

Bulgur Chickpea Salad

Bulgur, a whole grain, is the main ingredient in this quick side dish. With the addition of the chickpeas, this dish is high in dietary fiber. This recipe was adapted from *Making It Fit: Piecing Together Your Food Needs*, University of Vermont Extension, September 1998.

Serves 6

1¼ cups water
1 cup coarse bulgur
1 teaspoon dried parsley
1 teaspoon dried minced onion or use 1 tablespoon fresh chopped
   onion
1 teaspoon soy sauce (reduced sodium)
½ cup chopped scallions (green onions)
½ cup raisins
½ cup chopped carrots
1 (15 oz.) can chickpeas, drained and rinsed

Dressing
2 tablespoons olive or canola oil
2 tablespoons lemon juice
1 tablespoon soy sauce (reduced sodium)
1 garlic clove, minced
Black pepper, to taste

Bring water to boil in medium saucepan. Stir in bulgur, parsley, minced onion, and soy sauce. Cover and reduce heat; simmer 10–20 minutes until all water is absorbed and bulgur is not too crunchy. Do not overcook. Remove from heat and cool; fluff with a fork.

Combine dressing ingredients; stir well. Pour over cooked bulgur and mix well. Stir in scallions, raisins, carrots, and chickpeas. Cover and chill several hours. Store in the refrigerator.

Jules' Summer Sauce for Pasta

Serves 4

6 ripe medium-sized tomatoes, finely chopped
2 cups (8 ounces) sliced mushrooms
6–8 ounces mozzarella cheese (fresh mozzarella is best), shredded
   or grated
½ cup chopped fresh basil
2 garlic gloves, minced
½ cup olive oil
1 teaspoon salt
1 pound spaghetti or linguine
½ cup Pecorino Romano cheese

Mix all ingredients together in a bowl and let stand for 1 hour at room temperature. Cook pasta; drain. Pour sauce on hot noodles and sprinkle with cheese.

Lynne's Best Tomato Sauce

There are two types of tomato sauce, those made from fresh tomatoes and those made from canned. Both are good. The fresh kind is especially good in the late summer when local tomatoes are plentiful and cheap. Either type can be made with additional vegetables.

Canned
1 yellow onion, finely chopped
4 cloves garlic, finely chopped
½ cup olive oil
2 (12 oz.) cans diced tomatoes (I like Muir Glen® with basil)
2 tablespoons oregano
5 bay leaves, crumbled
2 tablespoons basil
Salt, pepper, and splash of red wine, to taste

Meat option
2 each sweet and hot Italian sausages (or 1 lb. ground meat)
1 yellow onion, finely chopped
4 cloves garlic, finely chopped
2 cans diced tomatoes (I like Muir Glen® with basil)
2 tablespoons oregano
5 bay leaves, crumbled
2 tablespoons basil
Salt, pepper, and splash of red wine, to taste

Fresh
4 cloves garlic, finely chopped
¼ cup pine nuts or 12 stalks asparagus (break off the bottoms and
    chop into ½-inch chunks), optional
½ cup olive oil
2–3 fresh tomatoes, diced
2 tablespoons oregano
5 bay leaves, crumbled
2 tablespoons basil
Salt, pepper, and splash of red wine, to taste

Canned

Sauté the onion and garlic in oil on medium heat until translucent, then add tomatoes and turn down heat. (Tomato sauce has a very low boiling point.) Add spices and let simmer. The longer it cooks, the better it tastes.

Meat Option

Sauté meat until cooked, pour off most of the fat, then add onions and garlic and continue to sauté. Follow remaining instructions for the canned option above.

Fresh

Sauté the garlic and pine nuts or asparagus (if using) in oil on medium heat, then add tomatoes, wine, and spice, and let simmer until the sauce thickens through evaporation.

If you like, you can add extra vegetables (such as mushrooms, peppers, and carrots) at the end of the onion step.

Sauce will keep in your fridge for about a week or can be frozen in a canning jar if you have extra (just make sure you leave some room in the jar for freezing expansion and let it cool before you stick it in the freezer).

Grasso's Sautéed Kale

Serves 6

2 large bunches fresh kale (preferably from your garden)
1 large red onion
4 cloves minced garlic
4 tablespoons olive oil
1 tablespoon balsamic vinegar
1 tablespoon water

Rinse kale bunches. Chop the leaf portion loosely, and cut the stems into ½-inch lengths.

Leave the kale in a colander in your sink while you prepare the other ingredients. (Note: you can sprinkle with lemon juice beforehand to further enhance the beneficial phytonutrients found in this vegetable; in fact, I always have lemon in my kitchen to sprinkle on fresh fruits and vegetables while I cook as it not only enhances the benefits but also keeps them from turning brown.)

Preheat large cast-iron frying pan with olive oil.

Add garlic and sauté quickly until the garlic turns a tan color.

Add chopped red onion and sauté a few more minutes. Add the chopped kale (it seems like a lot of kale, but don't worry, it shrinks down quickly, so you can add in batches if your skillet is too small) and stir briskly as it cooks, coating the kale in the oil-garlic-onion mix.

Once the kale is darker and turning limp, add the balsamic vinegar and stir, quickly add the water and cover to steam the whole dish (the kale absorbs the flavors this way).

Serve hot as a side dish for most any meal. Kids love this dish, too and kale is widely recognized as being a great detoxification food and one of the healthiest of vegetables. One thing to note—the way I like to cook kale, via my friend Tom Grasso, is not "quite" as healthy as steaming where the fiber does some beneficial binding, but it is just so delicious cooked this way and it is still beneficial.

Favorite Steamed Carrots

Serves 4

5–6 carrots, scrubbed with a brush under cold running water (if not
  organic, you should peel them)
1 tablespoon brown sugar
Canola margarine

Melt margarine in a saucepan under medium heat. Add carrots
and sauté until tender (about 5–10 minutes). Add brown sugar and
sauté a bit more.

Serve as a delicious side dish, hot or cold.

> You can make this dish even healthier if you steam the carrots first and
> then quickly add them to the frying pan.

Lynne's Summer Salad

Serves 4

Dressing
1 cup olive oil
⅓ cup red, balsamic, or red wine vinegar
⅓ cup white balsamic vinegar
2 teaspoons honey mustard or Dijon mustard
Pinch of salt
Pinch of freshly ground pepper
1 tablespoon finely chopped shallots (optional) or 2 cloves garlic, finely chopped

Salad
3 cups fresh greens or 1 head lettuce
2–4 carrots, peeled and chopped
¾ cup red cabbage
¼ cup finely chopped red onion
1 avocado, diced
Cucumber, mushrooms, red peppers, sesame seeds, garbanzo beans (optional)

Dressing
Take a canning jar or an old olive oil glass container, and add ingredients in order. Once everything is in the glass jar, seal it with the top and give it a few shakes. It is always nice to lightly dress a salad before serving, if you think you have the right amount, but that should be done right before serving so it doesn't get too heavy with the oil.

Salad

Wash lettuce well and use a spinner to dry, or wrap in dish towel and spin yourself (ideally outside, so you don't spray water). Add additional vegetables, dressing, and serve.

> Other good additions for this salad include arugula, endive, and cilantro.
>
> My friend, Lynne, is a master gardener. I love going to her house to sit in her kitchen on a late summer's day and chop vegetables with other friends to make this wonderful, colorful salad—right out of her garden. We also sip a nice red wine when we do this. According to Dr. Wayne Andersen (and other doctors from the Mayo Clinic), there is something in red wine that appears to help your heart. It's possible that antioxidants, such as flavonoids or a substance called resveratrol, have heart-healthy benefits. While drinking too much alcohol can have harmful effects on your body, a glass now and then may actually be beneficial!

Tuna and Beet Greens

Serves 4

4–5 cups baby beet greens
1 scallion, chopped
1 (5 oz.) can chunk light tuna fish
¼ cup garlic and peppercorn salad dressing (more or less to taste)

Place greens on individual plates. Sprinkle with scallions. Top with a dollop of tuna fish and drizzle with salad dressing and serve.

Broccoli Rice with White Bean Sauce

1 cup cannellini or white Northern beans, cooked,
   or 1 (10 oz.) can, drained, and heat to serving temperature
1 clove garlic, minced
½ cup Parmesan cheese
1 ½ cup brown rice, cooked
1 cup broccoli, steamed

Blend warmed beans with garlic and add the Parmesan cheese.
Serve over hot rice and broccoli.

Tiger Balls

1 cup peanut butter or almond butter
2-4 tablespoons honey
¼ cup raisins, finely chopped
2–4 tablespoons non-instant milk powder
4 tablespoons nutritional yeast
1 tablespoon oats (optional)
1 tablespoon coconut flour (optional)
¼ cup unsweetened shredded coconut

Mix nut butter and honey together. Add raisins. Add small
amounts of milk powder, nutritional yeast, instant oats and/or
coconut flour to stiffen mixture enough so that it can be formed
into balls. (Amounts may vary according to the variety or brand of
nut butter.) Form with hands into balls about 1-inch in diameter
and roll in coconut. Makes approximately 20 balls.

Almond Miso Spread

Almond butter, to taste
White miso, to taste

Spread equal amounts on bread or rice cake for a sandwich.

> Make this similar to how you would a peanut butter and jelly sandwich.
> It's a hearty and tasty variation.

Chocolate Almond Spread

Almond butter, to taste
Honey, to taste
Cocoa powder, to taste

Mix and adjust quantities to taste, and spread on bread or rice cakes for an easy treat.

Carolyn's Sweet Sesame Spread

⅔ cup tahini
⅓ cup honey
½ cup sesame seeds, blended slightly but still crunchy

Stir tahini and honey together in small mixing bowl. Add seeds to thicken and make crunchy, but still spreadable.

Spread 1-2 tablespoons on bread or rice cakes.

Tastes like halvah candy!

Desserts

Vanilla Cake

(As seen in *Living with Crohn's and Colitis* by Dede Cummings and Jessica Black, N.D.)

Serves 6

¾ cup organic butter or 1 cup coconut oil
3½ cups all-purpose gluten-free baking flour
1¼ cup honey
4 large hormone-free eggs
2 teaspoons vanilla extract
1 tablespoon plus 1 teaspoon baking powder
1 teaspoon baking soda
1 teaspoon xanthan gum
1 teaspoon salt
1½ cups almond milk

Preheat oven to 350°F. Lightly oil two 8- to 9-inch round cake pans and dust with gluten-free flour. Melt butter or coconut oil and beat with honey until it becomes fluffy. Lower the speed and add the eggs one at a time while beating. Add vanilla.

In a separate bowl, sift together all dry ingredients. Add half the dry mixture to the wet mixture and beat on low speed until combined. Then add the remaining half of the dry ingredients and beat on low speed until smooth. Add the almond milk to fold into the batter with a spoon.

Divide batter equally between the two prepared pans. Bake in preheated oven for 35–40 minutes or until a fork can be inserted and comes out clean. Cool the cake for 20 minutes in the pans. Insert a knife around the entire edge loosening the cake from the sides of the pan. Then turn cake over onto wire racks, being very careful when easing the cake out of the pan. Cool completely before frosting.

The two cake layers can be layered on top of each other with or without frosting or filling between the layers.

Honey Vanilla Frosting

(As seen in *Living with Crohn's and Colitis* by Dede Cummings and Jessica Black, N.D.)

3 egg whites
⅔ cup honey
Pinch of salt
½ teaspoon xanthan gum
1 teaspoon vanilla

Put the unbeaten egg whites, honey, xanthan gum, and salt into the top of a double boiler over hot water. Beat with an electric beater on medium to high speed, while you bring the water to a boil. Continue to beat for 7 minutes, or until the mixture forms soft mounds. Remove from the heat, add the vanilla slowly and continue beating until frosting is stiff enough to hold its shape. Wait for the frosting to cool before frosting.

Almond Cake with Banana, Coconut, and Pineapple Puree

(As seen in *Living with Crohn's and Colitis* by Dede Cummings and Jessica Black, N.D.)

Serves 6

2 eggs
4 tablespoons honey
3 over-ripe bananas, peeled
½ teaspoon baking powder
2¾ cups almond meal
Juice of ½ lemon
1 teaspoon vanilla extract
2 cups chopped pineapple
½ cup shredded coconut
1 ripe banana

Preheat the oven to 350°F. Generously grease a 9-inch round pie pan. Beat eggs and honey for 10 minutes or until pale and fluffy, then use a fork to mash the 3 over-ripe bananas into this mixture. Add ground almonds and baking powder and stir well. Lastly, stir in the lemon juice and vanilla. Mix until all lumps are dissolved.

Pour into baking pan and bake for 45 minutes or until golden brown on the outside and fork inserted in the middle comes out clean. Remove from the oven and leave in pan on a wire rack until completely cooled.

While cooling, add chopped pineapple, coconut, and banana to blender and blend until smooth. Once cooled, insert knife around all edges to loosen the cake. Invert cake quickly onto a flat plate and ease cake out of the pan. Cover with pureed mixture and top with fruit to make a flower decoration.

Coconut Macaroons

(As seen in *Living with Crohn's and Colitis* by Dede Cummings and Jessica Black, N.D.)

Serves 8

3 cups unsweetened, dried coconut flakes
1 cup almond meal
½ cup raw cacao powder or carob powder (see note)
½ cup maple syrup
¼ cup organic coconut butter
1 teaspoon organic vanilla extract
Pinch of Himalayan or sea salt

Mix all ingredients together and roll into balls. For a raw dessert, place in dehydrator and dehydrate for 24 hours at a low temperature.

To bake, place on greased cookie sheet and bake at 350°F for 8–10 minutes.

If you don't want to use cacao or carob, you can substitute with another ½ cup of almond meal or coconut.

Chewy Maple Granola Squares

Makes 15–30 squares

3 cups uncooked oatmeal (either old-fashioned or instant)
1 cup wheat germ
1 cup shredded coconut
½ cup all-bran cereal
1 cup raisins
¼ cup melted butter or margarine
⅔ cup light brown sugar
⅔ cup pure Vermont maple syrup
1 teaspoon vanilla

In a large bowl, combine the oatmeal, wheat germ, coconut, all-bran cereal, and raisins. Mix well, and set aside.

In a microwave-safe bowl, melt the butter or margarine for about 30 seconds. To the melted butter, add brown sugar, maple syrup, and vanilla. Mix well.

Combine the dry ingredients with the wet ingredients and mix well. You want to make sure that all the dry ingredients are covered with the syrup mixture.

Preheat oven to 375°F. Press mixture into a 9-inch x 13-inch pan that has been sprayed with cooking spray. Bake for 15–20 minutes, or until it is lightly browned.

Cool before cutting into squares or bars.

Bran Muffins

Makes 2–3 dozen

3 cups buttermilk
3 cups bran
1 cup oil (or ½ cup butter)
3 eggs
1 cup white sugar
1 cup brown sugar
1 teaspoon vanilla
3 teaspoons baking soda
2 teaspoons salt
1 cup raisins
3 cups flour
3 teaspoons baking powder

Preheat oven to 325°F. Mix buttermilk and bran and let stand. Mix oil, eggs, and sugars. Add vanilla, baking soda, salt, and raisins. Combine flour and baking powder. Combine bran mixture with liquid mixture. Quickly add flour mixture. Bake for 25–30 minutes.

Trina's Gluten-Free Apple Crisp

Serves 8

1 cup oat flour
1 cup oats
1 cup brown sugar
1 teaspoon cinnamon
½ cup margarine or butter, cold and diced
8 cup cored, peeled, sliced apples

Preheat oven to 375°F.

Mix first 4 ingredients, and cut in margarine with a fork to a crumbly consistency. Place apples in greased baking dish, then spread oat mixture on top. Bake for 1 hour, or until bubbly and crispy.

Joan's Chocolate Mousse with Raspberry Sauce

Serves 6

Mousse
12 ounces dark-chocolate chips (organic)
12 ounces silken extra-firm tofu
Pinch salt
½ cup brown sugar and/or 1 teaspoon vanilla (optional)

Sauce
10 ounces frozen raspberries (organic)
¼ cup brown sugar (optional)

Mousse
In double boiler, melt chocolate. In blender, blend tofu, salt, and optional ingredients. Add hot melted chocolate. Blend until smooth. Chill at least one hour before serving.

Sauce
Mix sugar and berries. Let stand 30 minutes before serving over chocolate mousse.

Blueberry Crumb Cake

Serves 9

Cake
1 cup all-purpose flour
½ cup granulated sucralose
2 teaspoons baking powder
¼ teaspoon salt
1 large egg
½ cup skim milk
1 tablespoon canola oil
½ teaspoon vanilla extract
1 cup blueberries (fresh or frozen)

Topping
6 tablespoons all-purpose flour
3 tablespoons granulated sucralose
2 tablespoons margarine
Nonstick spray

Preheat oven to 375°F. Spray an 8-inch × 8-inch baking pan with nonstick spray.

In a bowl, whisk together the flour, sucralose, baking powder, and salt. In another bowl, combine the egg, milk, canola oil, and vanilla extract. Stir wet mixture into dry mixture, mixing until just combined.

Pour batter into prepared pan. Sprinkle blueberries over the batter.

To make topping, combine flour and sucralose in a small bowl. Cut in margarine until mixture resembles coarse crumbs. Sprinkle topping evenly over blueberries. Bake for 35–45 minutes until edges of cake pull away from sides of the pan.

Let cool and cut into 9 pieces.

Fresh Fruit Tarts

Serves 12

12 wonton skins
2 tablespoons sugar-free jelly or fruit spread
1½ cup diced fresh fruit (see note)
1 cup non-fat yogurt, any flavor
Nonstick spray

Preheat oven to 375°F and spray muffin tins with cooking spray. Press wonton skins into muffin tins allowing the corners to stand up over the edges. Bake wontons until lightly brown. Watch carefully, wonton skins may cook very quickly. Remove from oven and carefully take each wonton out of the muffin tin and allow time for cooling.

   Warm jelly or fruit spread and lightly coat bottom of each wonton. Fill each bowl with fruit and a rounded dollop of yogurt on top. Garnish with small piece of fruit or a dab of jelly and serve immediately.

Fruit combinations depend on what is in season. Any of the following could be used: bananas, strawberries, blueberries, grapes, kiwi, raspberries, peaches, orange sections, etc.

This recipe can be used as a dessert or as an appetizer. It is very easy to prepare and looks lovely. Wonton shells are generally located near the produce section in the grocery store and do not need to be refrigerated until after they are opened. The baked wonton shells could also be filled with pudding, ice cream or other dessert-type items. They could also be used as a luncheon dish by filling them with chicken, tuna, or crab salad.

Buttermilk Chocolate Cake

Serves 6–8

1¾ cups all-purpose flour
½ cup plus 2 tablespoons sucralose, brown sugar blend
¾ cup cocoa powder
1½ teaspoons baking soda
1½ teaspoons baking powder
2 teaspoons cinnamon
¼ teaspoon salt
1¼ cups 1-percent buttermilk
2 large eggs
¼ cup tub margarine (not light), melted
1½ teaspoons vanilla extract
1 cup boiling water
Nonstick spray
Powdered sugar for garnish (optional)

Preheat oven to 350°F. Coat a 9- × 13-inch baking dish with nonstick spray. In a large bowl, combine flour, brown-sugar blend sucralose, cocoa, baking soda, baking powder, cinnamon, and salt. Set aside.

In a large mixing bowl, combine buttermilk, eggs, melted margarine, and vanilla. Mix on low speed until well blended. Gradually beat in boiling water. Gradually add flour mixture and mix on low speed until just blended. Pour batter into prepared pan, and bake 25 minutes or until a toothpick inserted in center comes out clean.

Cool cake on a wire rack. Dust with powdered sugar if desired.

Banana Pineapple Delight

Serves 16

1½ cups graham cracker crumbs
⅓ cup reduced-fat margarine
2 bananas
1 (8 oz.) package reduced-fat cream cheese (or Neufchatel), softened
1½ cups skim milk
1 package (four servings) sugar-free, instant vanilla pudding
1 (20 oz.) can crushed pineapple, drained
4 ounces frozen lite whipped topping, thawed

Mix graham cracker crumbs and reduced-fat margarine with fork or pastry cutter until margarine is cut into crumbs. Wet fingers and press mixture into bottom of a 9-inch x 13-inch baking dish. No baking is required. Slice bananas and spread evenly over crumb mixture.

Beat softened cream cheese until very smooth and gradually add milk, beating until smooth. Add pudding mix, and beat 1 minute or until mixture begins to thicken. Spoon evenly over bananas and spread with rubber scraper. Spread drained, crushed pineapple over the pudding layer. Spread whipped topping over pineapple layer with rubber scraper, making sure to spread to edges of baking dish. Refrigerate for at least one hour, but refrigerating for three or more hours is best. Cut into 16 pieces and serve chilled.

Orange Poppy Seed Cake

Serves 8

Cake

1½ cups granulated sucralose
3 large eggs
1⅓ cups cottage cheese (4% fat)
1 cup fat-free plain yogurt
⅓ cup canola oil
4½ tablespoons frozen orange juice concentrate, thawed
1½ tablespoons finely grated orange rind
2 cups all-purpose flour
3½ teaspoons baking powder
3 teaspoons poppy seeds
¾ teaspoon baking soda
Nonstick spray

Glaze

1 ounce light cream cheese, softened
½ cup powdered sugar
1½ tablespoons frozen orange juice concentrate, thawed

Cake

Preheat the oven to 350°F. Spray a 9- ×13-inch pan with nonstick spray.

In a large bowl, combine sucralose, eggs, and cottage cheese. Beat on high speed of electric mixer until smooth. Add yogurt, oil, orange juice concentrate, and orange rind. Continue beating until smooth.

In another bowl, combine flour, baking powder, poppy seeds, and baking soda. Stir the dry ingredients into the orange mixture until everything is just combined. Pour the mixture into prepared pan.

Place the pan in the center of the oven and bake for 25–30 minutes or until a tester inserted in the center comes out clean. Cool on a wire rack.

Glaze

In a small mixing bowl, combine all ingredients for glaze. Beat on medium speed of an electric mixer until smooth. Spread glaze evenly over cake.

Fast Fruit Salad or Dessert

Serves 8

1 (8 oz.) can pineapple tidbits in light juice, drained well
1 (8 oz.) can chunky mixed fruit in light juice, drained well
1 (11 oz.) can mandarin oranges, in light juice, drained well
1 cup grapes, white, red, or mixed, cut in half
1 cup reduced-fat sour cream
2 tablespoons granulated sucralose
¼ cup flaked coconut (optional)

Combine all ingredients in a medium-sized serving bowl. Garnish with flaked coconut, if desired. Serve immediately or chill until time to serve.

Peach and Berry Crisp

Serves 16

6 cups fresh or frozen sliced peaches, peeled and drained
2 cups fresh or frozen blueberries, raspberries, or blackberries
3–4 tablespoons granulated sucralose
½ teaspoon ground nutmeg
¼ teaspoon cinnamon
½ cup oatmeal
4 tablespoons flour
2 tablespoons packed brown sugar
2 tablespoons reduced-calorie margarine
¼ teaspoon cinnamon

Preheat oven to 375°F. Combine peaches and berries in an ungreased 11- x 7-inch inch baking pan. Mix sucralose, nutmeg, and cinnamon in small bowl, sprinkle over fruit, and stir gently.

Mix oatmeal, flour, brown sugar, margarine, and cinnamon together and spread over fruit.

Bake, uncovered, 35–40 minutes.

Special Amazing Secret Creamy Sauce with Berries

Blueberries
Raspberries
Any other berries of your choice, a handful of each
1 cup raw cashews
1–2 cups almond milk
⅓ cup fresh orange juice
A little agave nectar (or honey or maple syrup)

Cover the cashews with an inch of water and soak for 1–2 hours.

Drain cashews and transfer them to a blender (I love using my Vitamix® blender).

Add almond milk, orange juice, and agave. Blend.

Add more almond milk to obtain desired creaminess and add more orange juice for an extra zing.

Spoon the cream over the berries and go to heaven.

My sister, Alex, says, "I like my cashew cream to be quite thick, like ice cream. If you add about one cup of ice to this recipe, it will actually turn into nut ice cream."

Johanna's Blueberry-Lime Coconut Cake

Serves 4–6

⅓ cup butter
1 cup light brown sugar
6 eggs
1 teaspoon vanilla
½ cup Let's Do . . . Organic® coconut flour
¼ cup ground almonds
¼ cup lime juice
Zest of one lime
1 cup blueberries

Grease an 8- x 10-inch baking pan and flour with coconut flour or with sugar for a slightly crunchy bottom. Preheat oven to 350°F.

Cream the butter and sugar. Add the eggs and vanilla, then add the coconut flour and almonds. Add the lime juice and zest, then gently fold in the blueberries.

Pour the batter into the greased and floured pan.

Decorate with very thin pieces of lime.

Bake for 30 minutes.

> For an extra zesty flavor, you can combine confectioner's sugar and lemon or lime juice and frost the top of the cake once it has cooled.

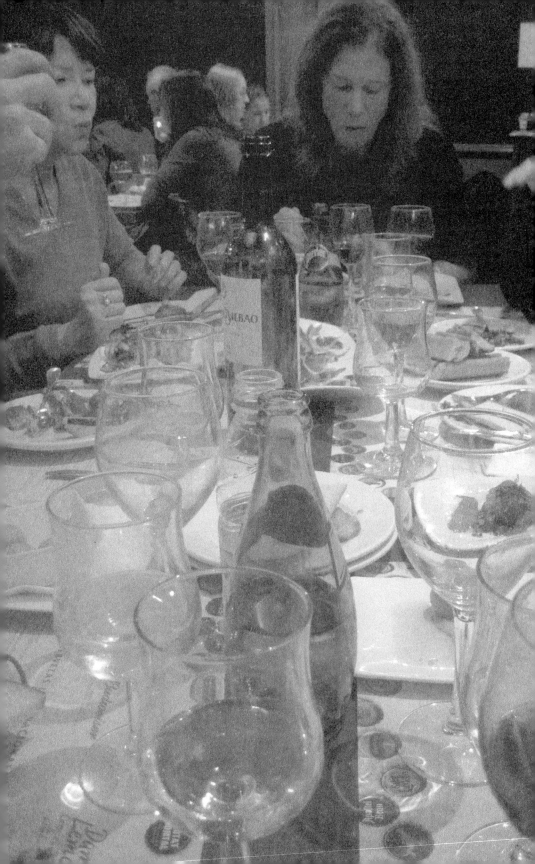

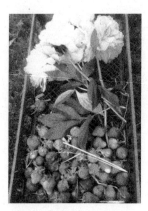

Food Substitution
Chart for Cooking
and Baking

Substitutions Chart

Eliminated Food	Substitution	Directions
Cow's milk	Soy milk, rice milk, sesame seed milk, almond milk (or other nut milk), oat milk	Substitute equal quantities
Commercial eggs	Organic eggs are fine for some individuals. Or you can experiment with some of the following binders:	
	Flaxseeds soaked overnight in water or boiled for 15 minutes	1–2 tablespoons seeds in ½–1 cup of water
	Tofu, for scrambles or baked goods	¼ cup in place of 1 egg
	Banana, to bind baked goods (adds a sweet taste)	½–1 banana in cookies or muffins
	Arrowroot powder (use as a binder for nongluten flours)	1 tablespoon for each cup of nongluten flour
	Guar gum (you need only a very small amount)	¼–½ teaspoon for muffins, breads, and other baked goods
	Xantham gum	1 teaspoon for each cup of non-gluten flour
Sugar	Honey (twice as sweet as processed cane sugar)	½ amount recipe calls for
	Pure maple syrup	½–¾ amount recipe calls for
	Brown rice syrup	½–¾ amount recipe calls for
	Stevia	Small amount; label will have conversions

Eliminated Food	Substitution	Directions
Wheat flour	When substituting these flours, you may want to add a little more baking powder or baking soda to help the baked goods rise.	
	Amaranth (can have a strong taste)	Needs a binder (see above)
	Barley (contains a small amount of gluten)	May need a binder
	Garbanzo	Needs a binder
	Kamut (contains gluten; should not be eaten every day)	No binder is needed
	Oat (may contain a very small amount of gluten)	May need a binder
	Quinoa (can taste bitter; should be mixed with other flours)	Needs a binder
	Rice (can be grainy; mix with other flours)	Needs a binder
	Rye (contains gluten; should not be eaten every day)	No binder is needed
	Soy (can have a beany flavor)	Needs a binder
	Spelt (contains gluten; should not be eaten every day)	No binder is needed
	Teff	Needs a binder
Potatoes	Yucca root, taro root, Jerusalem artichokes (sunchokes)	Cook similar to potatoes
Chocolate	Carob powder is nutritionally superior to chocolate	Substitute 3 tablespoons for 1 ounce chocolate
Butter	Blend of organic butter and olive oil (use as a spread) Blend of organic butter and coconut oil (use for baking) Nonhydrogenated vegan margarine spread	Substitute equal quantities
Peanuts, peanut butter	Almonds, almond butter	Substitute equal quantities

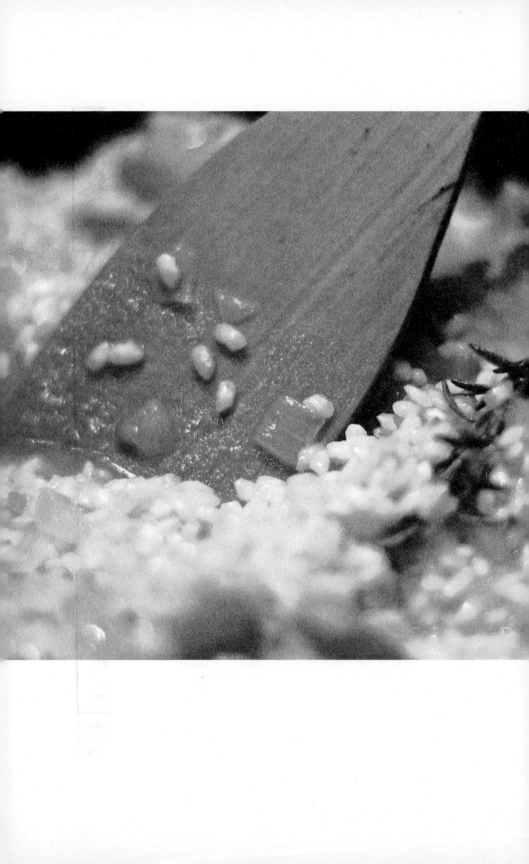

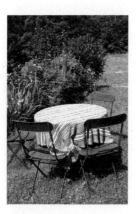

References

References

Online Resources

The Crohn's & Colitis Foundation of America
www.ccfa.org
A non-profit, volunteer-driven organization dedicated to finding the cure for Crohn's disease and ulcerative colitis.

Epicurious
www.epicurious.com
A great resource for cooks-on-the-go, and ones who like to use their smart phones, or iPhones/iPads in the kitchen!

Gluten Free Help
http://glutenfreehelp.info

HealingWell
www.healingwell.com
Social network and support community. You'll find information, resources, and support, plus full access to the forums and chat rooms.

Healthline
www.healthline.com

Healthy Children
www.healthychildren.org

Ideas Kids: Resources for Children and Teens with Intestinal Disease
www.ideaskids.com/teens/teenssupport.html

I Have UC
www.ihaveuc.com
My friend, Adam, started this site a few years ago and he started one for me called www.ihavecrohns.com. Adam is amazing with social-networking and is an overall great guy who has supported me and countless other ulcerative colitis patients worldwide with his wit, sense of humor, and compassion. Check this site out for sure!

Irritable Bowel Syndrome Health Center
www.webmd.com/ibs/default.htm

Mayo Clinic
www.mayoclinic.com

National Digestive Diseases Information Clearinghouse
digestive.niddk.nih.gov/index.htm

The Organic Center
www.organic-center.org

Sodastream Pure Soda Maker
www.sodastreamusa.com
It's quick and easy. You'll save on lugging, storing, and disposing of bottles and cans of store-bought soda. You can fizz and flavor to your taste, without high-fructose corn syrup or aspartame.

Vitamix®
www.vitamix.com
Vitamix® has been manufacturing high-performance blending equipment for over 85 years.

Books and Other Resources

Andersen Wayne Scott, *Dr. A's Habits of Health: The Path to Permanent Weight Control and Optimal Health*, Habits of Health Press, 2009.
Dr. Andersen's book has so much useful information about diet and lifestyle support, plus he has an informative website and e-mail newsletters with useful, weekly tips.

Black, Jessica K., N.D., *The Anti-Inflammation Diet and Recipe Book: Protect Yourself and Your Family from Heart Disease, Arthritis, Diabetes, Allergies, and More*, Hunter House, 2006.
This book offers excellent recipes that are completely hypoallergenic and anti-inflammatory.

References

D'Adamo, Peter and Catherine Whitney, *Eat Right for Your Type*, Putnam, 1996.
For individuals who do not know what they are intolerant to, or for those extra sensitive individuals who seem to react to odd foods that are not termed "inflammatory," other diets might be an option. The *Eat Right for Your Type* diet was developed by Dr. Peter D'Adamo. He scientifically and elegantly describes how certain foods are better tolerated or more aggravating for an individual depending on that person's blood type. He further discusses particular foods that may be a benefit for some blood types, but can be hindering for others. He describes foods, types of exercises, and even condiments and seasonings that are more appropriate for individuals based on their blood type.

Eden, Donna, *Energy Medicine: Balancing Your Body's Energies for Optimal Health, Joy, and Vitality*, Tarcher, 2008.
This is such an excellent book and it can offer many ideas on daily tapping routines to increase the flow of energy in the body and help to make healing possible.

Fallon, Sally, *Nourishing Traditions: The Cookbook that Challenges Politically Correct Nutrition and the Diet Dictocrats*, New Trends Publishing, 1999.
This is a cookbook and an excellent resource if you want to learn how to begin making more homemade fermented foods.

Gates, Donna and Linda Schatz, *The Body Ecology Diet: Recovering Your Health and Rebuilding Your Immunity*, Body Ecology, 2006.
This book discusses increasing gastrointestinal resistance and overall health by the use of probiotics.

Gershon, Michael D., *Second Brain: The Scientific Basis of Gut Instinct and a Groundbreaking New Understanding: of Nervous Disorders of the Stomach and Intestine*, Harper-Collins, 1998.
A book that explores the enteric nervous system, otherwise known as the brain of the gut, sometimes with humor.

Gottschall, Elaine Gloria, *Breaking the Vicious Cycle: Intestinal Health Through Diet*, Kirkton Press, 1994.
Investigates the link between food and intestinal disorders such as Crohn's disease, ulcerative colitis, diverticulitis, celiac disease, cystic fibrosis, and chronic diarrhea.

Kamm, Laura Alden, *Intuitive Wellness: Using Your Body's Inner Wisdom to Heal*, Atria Books/Beyond Words, 2006.
Laura Alden Kamm endured her own personal health journey and came out on the "other side" in her remarkable memoir.

Kinderlehrer, Jane, *Confessions of a Sneaky Organic Cook or, How to Make Your Family Healthy When They're Not Looking!*, New American Library, 1972.
This is an older book but has so many good ideas in it.

Lair, Cythia, *Feeding the Whole Family: Cooking with Whole Foods*, Sasquatch Books, 2008.
This is a fun book that gives many ideas on quick meals for the family.

Remen, Rachel Naomi, M.D., *Kitchen Table Wisdom: Stories that Heal*, Riverhead Trade Books, 1997.
Remen is one of a growing number of physicians exploring the spiritual dimension of the healing arts.

Santorelli, Saki, *Heal Thy Self: Lessons on Mindfulness in Medicine*, Three Rivers Press, 2000.
Santorelli, director of the Stress Reduction Clinic at the University of Massachusetts Medical Center, does a wonderful job with this book and it is one of Dede's favorites in aiding her recovery. Santorelli guides the reader through the process of learning to listen to our bodies, and bring mindfulness into our lives. Most of the patients in the Stress Reduction Clinic have never meditated, or been involved in groups or alternative therapies, so his work, and that of the clinic's founder, Jon Kabat-Zinn, is highly regarded and a model of success.

Scala, James, *The New Eating Right for a Bad Gut: The Complete Nutritional Guide to Ileitis, Colitis, Crohn's Disease, and Inflammatory Bowel Disease*, Plume, 2000.
Dr. Scala's book was one of Dede's first purchases at her local used bookstore after diagnosis. His advice and step-by-step dietary guidelines are enhanced by his clear and concise education in eating a healthy diet; a great compliment for a learning library.

References

Straus, Martha B., *No-Talk Therapy for Children and Adolescents,* by W.W. Norton, 1999.
Straus opens for readers a huge grab bag of gimmicks, gadgets, and games from which to draw resources appropriate to every no-talk occasion. This book will be useful for parents or caregivers of younger IBS patients who struggle with a lack of language with which to express their emotions.

Weil, Andrew, *8 Weeks to Optimum Health: A Proven Program for taking Full Advantage of Your Body's Natural Healing Power,* Ballantine Books, 2007.
Dr. Weil is one of our "health gurus" and, again, a great book and website resource.

Yee, Rodney. *A.M. and P.M. Yoga.* DVD. Director: Steve Adams. Rating: NR (not rated).

Yee, Rodney. *Moving Toward Balance: 8 weeks of Yoga with Rodney Yee,* Rodale Books, 2004.
Website: www.yeeyoga.com.
Rodney and his wife, Colleen Saidman, have been wonderful supporters of my writing and my yoga practice. I owe much of my health and well-being to them!

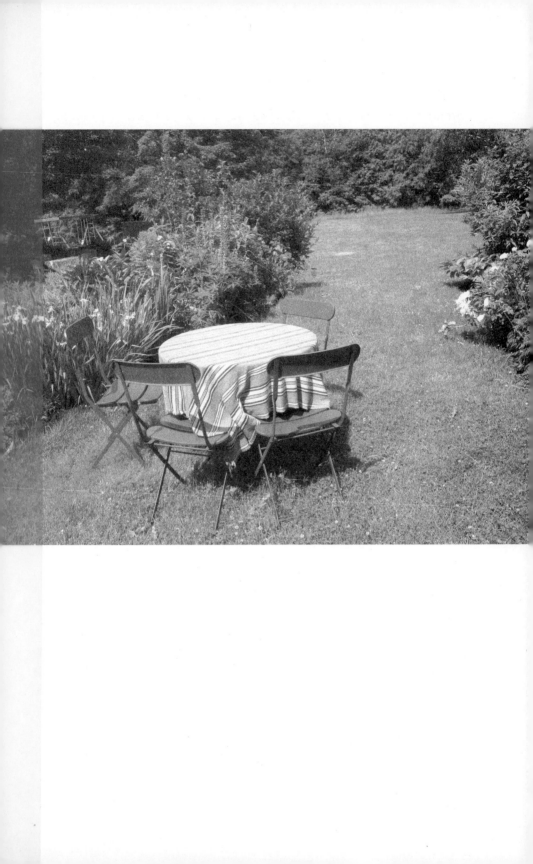

Also in the *Cooking Well* Series . . .

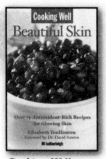

Cooking Well:
Beautiful Skin
978-1-57826-323-3

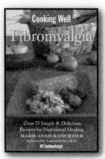

Cooking Well:
Fibromyalgia
978-1-57826-362-2

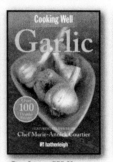

Cooking Well:
Garlic
978-1-57826-343-1

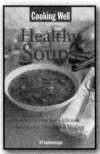

Cooking Well:
Healthy Soups
978-1-57826-371-4

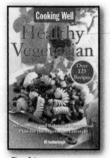

Cooking
Well: Healthy
Vegetarian
978-1-57826-389-9

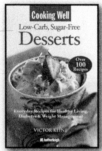

Cooking Well:
Low–Carb Sugar–
Free Desserts
978-1-57826-325-7

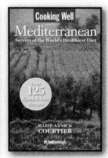

Cooking Well:
Mediterranean
978-1-57826-314-1

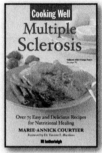

Cooking Well:
Multiple Sclerosis
978-1-57826-301-1

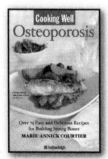

Cooking Well:
Osteoporosis
978-1-57826-302-8

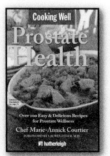

Cooking Well:
Prostate Health
978-1-57826-376-9

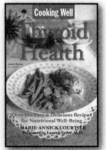

Cooking Well:
Thyroid Health
978-1-57826-352-3

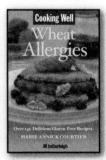

Cooking Well:
Wheat Allergies
978-1-57826-313-4

For more information on these and other Hatherleigh Press titles,
visit www.hatherleighpress.com.